OXFORD MEDICAL PUBLICATIONS

Cystic Fibrosis

THE FACTS

New edition

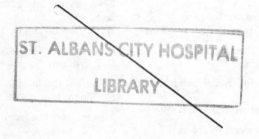

ALSO PUBLISHED BY OXFORD UNIVERSITY PRESS

Cystic Fibrosis

THE FACTS
New edition

ANN HARRIS
Lecturer in Molecular Genetics
United Medical and Dental Schools of
Guy's and St Thomas's Hospitals

and

MAURICE SUPER
Consultant Paediatric Geneticist, Royal
Manchester Children's Hospital

OXFORD NEW YORK TOKYO
OXFORD UNIVERSITY PRESS
1991

Oxford University Press, Walton Street, Oxford OX2 6DP

Oxford   New York   Toronto
Delhi   Bombay   Calcutta   Madras   Karachi
Petaling Jaya   Singapore   Hong Kong   Tokyo
Nairobi   Dar es Salaam   Cape Town
Melbourne   Auckland
and associated companies in
Berlin   Ibadan

Oxford is a trade mark of Oxford University Press

Published in the United States
by Oxford University Press, New York

British Library Cataloguing in Publication Data
Harris, Ann 1956–
Cystic fibrosis.-2nd ed.
1. Man. Pancreas. Cystic fibrosis
I. Title II. Super, Maurice III. Series
616.37
ISBN 0-19-262024-X   ISBN 0-19-262037-1 (Pbk)

Library of Congress Cataloging in Publication Data
Harris, Ann, 1956–
Cystic fibrosis : the facts / Ann Harris and Maurice Super. – 2nd ed.
(Oxford medical publications)
Includes index.
1. Cystic fibrosis in children—Popular works. I. Super,
Maurice. II. Title. III. Series.
RJ456.C9H37 1991   616.3'7—dc20   90-14272
ISBN 0-19-262024-X (hardback) ISBN 0-19-262037-1 (paperback)

Typeset by Downdell Limited, Oxford
Printed in Great Britain
by Biddles Ltd.
Guildford & King's Lynn

Acknowledgements

The authors would like to thank Mrs Georgina Briody, Miss Lynette Noble, Miss Elizabeth Manners and Miss Despina Savva for help with preparation of the original manuscript and figures.

We are grateful to Drs Sonja Gatzanis and Margaret Hodson, Clive Sandercock and Gary Gifford for helpful discussions and critical reading of parts of the manuscript.

Figure 3 was kindly provided by Dr R. Fraser Williams and Fig. 12 by the cytogenetics department of the Paediatric Research Unit, Guy's Hospital.

A.H. would like to thank Professor Paul E. Polani, who introduced her to the subject, and the Winston Churchill Memorial Trust.

M.S. thanks Dr Garry Hambleton for helpful discussions.

Preface to the second edition

Since the first edition of this book was written more than three years ago much has happened in the field of CF. The most important advance has been the isolation of the CF gene. This has had some immediate implications. However, more important will be the great increase in our understanding of the disease that will stem from now having the tool with which to ask fundamental questions about CF. It is impossible to speculate on how long it will take to translate these advances into better treatment for CF, but this will undoubtedly occur. The second edition of *Cystic Fibrosis—The Facts* is written at a time of great optimism, and we hope the text reflects that. The overall emphasis of the book has changed slightly in order to embrace up-to-date approaches to the management of CF, particular with respect to diet. New chapters on the psychology of CF and on heart–lung transplants in CF are included, and the research aspect of the disease becomes less prominent.

London and Manchester
April 1990

Contents

Introduction: living with cystic fibrosis

The needs of a child with cystic fibrosis (CF) change with age, but are generally much greater than those of a healthy child. Early on, the parents must help with regular physiotherapy, give medication, and pay special attention to increased dietary needs. They have to learn to tolerate a certain amount of illness in the child and to know when medical help or advice is needed. It is very easy for one or other parent, often the father, to 'opt out' of such decisions and to participate little in the child's treatment. The efficient CF clinic, operating an 'open door' policy, can help to make both parents part of the team and may defuse many of the inherent tensions associated with CF. Even so, both parents and the affected person have psychological ups and downs, sometimes feeling optimistic about the long-term outlook, sometimes pessimistic. The age at which a relative died of CF, or the death of a friend attending the CF clinic, may provide crisis points. Some adolescent rebellion against daily treatment may have its roots in gloominess at the long-term outlook. Some studies have shown that mothers of CF children become depressed from time to time, perhaps because they carry the main family burden of the illness.

For schoolchildren a persistent cough may be embarrassing and disrupt the class. Special arrangements may need to be made with the school to ensure that meals are sufficiently large. Affected children may be embarrassed at school by the large number of pancreatic enzyme capsules which they need to take with their meals. Pamphlets for teachers (e.g. 'Cystic Fibrosis and school', prepared by the CF Research Trust) may help the child's problems to be dealt with sympathetically, as may visits to the school by the CF nurse or dietician. Illness or treatment routines that include regular admission to hospital may result in the loss of many school days. Generally the child will be well enough to do at least some school work, and most children with CF manage to keep up remarkably well. Some older children have been attracted by ambulatory intravenous antibiotic treatment. This allows a greater degree of freedom, continued attendance at school, and the reassurance that the chronic chest infection is being kept under control. On the other hand, a short hospital admission for intravenous antibiotic treatment has the advantage that many aspects of the CF treatment can be checked at once.

Also, the CF team may become more aware of the needs of the child and family and can relieve the parents from the responsibility of physiotherapy for a short while. As the CF child becomes older, the parents may actually find the physiotherapy physically taxing. The forced expiration technique, described in the chapter on treatment of CF, may liberate them partly and provide the child with greater independence.

Adolescence brings its own problems. While it has become relatively easy to nourish younger affected children, some adolescents with CF lose weight or show a decline in their growth rate. As a result, more marked differences in their height and weight compared with their peers may come at an awkward time. Adolescent rebellion may result in loss of co-operation in taking medicines and having physiotherapy. At about 16 years of age we believe that there is benefit in transferring to the adult CF clinic, if one exists within a reasonable travelling distance. Being allowed to 'grow up' in this way may provide the stimulus to vigorous treatment once more.

An increasing number of CF patients is now reaching adulthood. In these competitive times adult CF sufferers may have to cope with unemployment, though many manage remarkably well in a wide variety of careers. Certain very physical occupations are closed to all but the most mildly affected. Men with CF will have to cope with almost certain sterility (though not impotence), and women need to remember the possible very adverse effect on health that a pregnancy may have, the physical hard work involved in caring for an infant, and the 1 in 50 or so risk they run of having an affected child.

LIVING WITH CYSTIC FIBROSIS

The following comments from members of families coping with CF are designed to give insight into the daily problems of living with this disease. First, the comments of 7-year-old Caroline who has taken the advice that she should learn to swim in order to have better lung function.

Cystic Fibrosis is alright. The only bad bit on my physiotherapy bed is that the surface scratches me. My mum has put some sheets over it so I don't mind any more. I like my mum doing the physiotherapy but I don't like the look of sputum. I don't like the Ventolin or the Ketovite liquid but I do like the salt tablets.

I do lots of exercise, cartwheels, hand-stands, flips, and forward and backward rolls. The best exercise is swimming. On Monday I go with the school and on Tuesday my mum takes me for swimming lessons. I am learning crawl, diving, swimming under water, and touching the bottom with my feet in the deep end.

Next, we have included the views of David, written 4 years ago when he was 13. David died in 1988 while waiting for a heart–lung transplant operation.

Being a child with CF isn't terrible, but it can be a bit of a pain in the neck. We try to be as normal as possible, but it can be quite difficult, with all the work involved.

Probably the worst thing used to be diet, children with CF find it difficult to put on weight. Now we can eat a normal diet, but we have to take a lot of enzyme capsules with each meal.

Another thing is physio. This has to be done twice per day, or if I have a cold or something like that, as many times as it needs to be cleared out. Physio isn't much fun if I'm in someone else's house watching videos or listening to records, because I always have to come home that bit sooner. School is quite normal. I go to an ordinary school and do everything that other children do. I have a lot of friends and get on with nearly everyone. You do get the odd wisecrack about your weight, but your either ignore them or give them a mouthful.

Every so often, I have to go into hospital for 10 days, which can be quite boring. In hospital, I am on intensive physio and i.v. [intravenous] treatment. Hospital isn't that bad, but when I get back to school I have quite a lot of work to copy up.

All together, CF is hard work, but it isn't as bad for me as it's made out to be.

David's mother's thoughts follow:

Being a parent of a CF child can be a demanding and very frustrating role. It affects you both mentally and physically. There isn't a moment of the day when CF is not in your thoughts. A routine has to be worked out, as everything revolves around these children. When you are told that your child has CF it is devastating, and when someone's child is ill all the other parents feel it and worry.

David is a very sensible and active 13-year-old, but he is susceptible to severe chest infections. If a cold is going around, he will catch it, and his normally twice a day physio will have to be stepped up, sometimes to every two hours, to keep on top of it. A cold can make him quite ill. Needless to say, both parent and child end up very tired and sometimes very argumentative. When David comes in a bit late, he does not want his physio done, and I don't feel like doing it. It would be very easy to say 'let's leave it', but it doesn't work that way and it's got to be done properly.

School causes quite a big problem, as there is always someone in the classroom who has got some infection to pass around; this is a constant worry. We have fortunately got a very understanding school, and the teachers have come to comprehend just what is wrong with David. Many parents have great difficulties in this area and for the children it can be a distressing situation. Being called 'skinny' isn't funny. David is with a grand set of lads who help him a lot and don't mind his coughs. One of the most intensely worrying times is when David is admitted to hospital. Having lost one boy with CF I dread the words 'X-ray' and what the doctors will tell me, but always strength seems to come from somewhere.

A doctor once asked me if he should paint the blackest picture to the parents. The answer is yes. The parent has to realize from the very start just what the situation is—the importance of the physio and an adequate diet and the consequences if these are not done.

Both parents have to pull together, and it isn't always easy. CF can either make you drift apart or pull you closer together. We are very fortunate.

CF children need a lot of time and attention, more so when they are not very well, and the mental strain is terrible. Bitterness does sometimes creep into it and you ask yourself, 'Why me?'. The answer is simple—I tell myself I'm special and have been given a very special child to look after.

Next, the comments of 17-year-old Dominic who, although healthy himself, has two younger brothers with CF.

Living with two brothers who suffer from cystic fibrosis can sometimes be very hard, but most of the time it isn't really that bad. I have to get up very early in the morning, at about 7.00 a.m., to help in the kitchen while the boys are having their physiotherapy. I don't really mind doing this, as I have got so used to it over the past few years, although I sometimes get irritable and argumentative over the slightest things.

I sometimes, rather selfishly, think that having physiotherapy is an excuse to miss out on helping with jobs around the house, but I have to realize that it cannot be helped if my brothers have cystic fibrosis. As physiotherapy is such an important part of their treatment, holidays may be slightly spoiled, over time allowed for going out during the day and at night, as it takes about half an hour for physio. It doesn't spoil all our holidays though, as we sometimes go to Lourdes, in France, to allow the boys to bathe in the waters and to pray for a cure, as well as being tourists.

Most of the time, I get on very well with my brothers, as they try to live normal lives, and I only hope that a cure for cystic fibrosis may soon come in the near future.

Overall, having to live with cystic fibrosis sufferers isn't really a big thing. We all manage to get on together as one big, happy family.

These comments by family members provide certain insights. We were able to reassure David's mother that he and other children with CF are not unduly susceptible to the mild infections of the schoolroom and that his immune system would cope with them quite normally without their causing deterioration of his CF. Many parents of younger children with CF need this reassurance to help prevent them mollycoddling the child. In David's mother's case her general worry about his advanced illness depressed her from time to time. When depression occurs it is generally the mother who shows it. David was exasperated by being undersized and about his illness in general, but not depressed.

Many older children with CF show denial of their disorder and its potential seriousness. This is a very common coping mechanism and is shared by many of the medical and paramedical members of the CF team. The latter need to be very positively oriented towards vigorous treatment but need to retain the insight that they may not always succeed.

Many of the psychological problems in CF spring from the unknown. It is difficult to face up to a disorder in which the long-term outlook for any individual may be impossible to predict. Some children go through a phase of repeated quite severe chest infections only to recover and stay well for years. Others do not recover or suffer the effects of permanent lung damage. There is always the hope of a miracle cure being discovered.

The infertility of males and the potential dangers of pregnancy in females contribute to fewer than average men and women with CF marrying. This said, people with CF do form lasting relationships.

The CF clinic, through the CF nurse, ward sister, physiotherapist, or dietician, plays a very important role in providing a listening ear and parents are encouraged to 'phone in with their queries or worries. In the beginning this may act as a crutch until self-confidence builds up. Life used to be more restricted for CF children. High doses of the newer enzymes allow the great majority to have no dietary restrictions at all. Energy needs are increased in CF, so more food than normal is needed, including protein and fat. Energetic dietary counselling may be needed to ensure that children and adolescents with CF continue to take sufficient food to satisfy the increased energy requirements. This is particularly so when fashion-conscious youngsters wish to be slim like their peers. Lethargy is an important danger sign and often signifies salt depletion. This occurs mainly but not exclusively in hot weather. It is quite easy to control, if thought of. Unexplained diarrhoea may signify a new chest infection rather than a dietary problem. So may a change in sputum colour, an increase in sputum or general irritability. They should all be reported to the doctor.

Except for neglecting physiotherapy and other CF treatment there are very few absolute 'don'ts' in CF.

This sketched outline of CF is elaborated on in the subsequent chapters.

1

What is cystic fibrosis?

Cystic fibrosis is an inherited disease that has its main effects on the digestive system and the lungs. It is usually diagnosed soon after birth, and symptoms occur throughout life. Nowadays, thanks to improvements in dietary supplements and better treatment, most people with cystic fibrosis can lead a fairly normal life. However, to achieve this they need daily treatment, consisting of chest physiotherapy, various medicines and pancreatic enzyme capsules taken with their food. In addition they have to pay special attention to their increased dietary needs.

The name cystic fibrosis (CF) describes the changes that occur at an early age in the pancreas of CF patients. (The pancreas is a major organ in the body, manufacturing digestive enzymes and other important compounds.) The part of the pancreas that produces digestive enzymes (proteins that digest food) is replaced by a characteristic fibrous scar tissue with fluid-filled spaces (cysts).

Another common feature of CF is unusually sticky or thick mucus secretions in the lungs and digestive system. In the lungs the presence of this thick or viscid mucus makes chest infections more severe. In the digestive system it may damage the pancreas, both directly and indirectly through blocking the ducts that form an open channel for digestive enzymes to reach the gut. This viscid mucus is the origin of another common name for CF: mucoviscidosis.

Until the beginning of this century doctors did not recognize CF as a disease in its own right. The various symptoms of CF were merely seen as separate, unrelated infections. Part of the reason for this was that before the advent of antibiotics, chest infections (which are a major feature of CF) were common in many diseases. The first recognition of CF came through another feature of the disease, namely steatorrhoea. Steatorrhoea means literally 'fatty stools', and is a condition characterized by the passage of pale, bulky, smelly faeces. Thus in 1912 the London physician Archibald Garrod described the occurrence of steatorrhoea in several members of the same family. The description, with hindsight, was almost certainly of CF.

The next clear description of CF came from a Swiss paediatrician named Fanconi. He described children with cystic fibrosis in 1928 and again in 1936. He also distinguished CF from coeliac disease, a disease caused by an inability to digest wheat proteins that has some symptoms in common with CF. When the initial descriptions of CF were made, there was some controversy as to whether steatorrhoea and recurrent attacks of severe bronchitis constituted a separate disease (both symptoms were common to several diseases in the pre-antibiotic era). It was not until other chest and digestive system diseases (e.g. pneumonia and bacillary dysentery) became treatable that this controversy was resolved.

It was found that in some cases treatment of chest or gut infections was ineffective, or gave only temporary relief. The patients unaffected by treatment were identified as CF sufferers. Thus Fanconi, working in Zurich, and Dorothy Anderson in Baltimore, were proved correct in recognizing CF as a specific disorder. A paper by Dorothy Anderson in 1938 gave an almost complete account of the development of CF, and a further paper in 1946 advocated treatment of the disease with a high-calorie, high-protein, low-fat diet supplemented with pancreatin (extract of animal pancreas). In 1948 Anderson and her co-worker Di'Santagnese confirmed another characteristic of the disease. They showed that CF patients are particularly prone to chest infections caused by *Staphylococcus* bacteria.

In 1952 there was a heatwave in New York. Perceptive physicians noted that the majority of children brought to casualty departments with heat prostration were CF sufferers. This led Di'Santagnese to the discovery of the greatly increased levels of salt in the sweat of people with CF. This has become the cornerstone on which the diagnosis of CF rests. A mother may notice a salty taste when she kisses her CF baby. Two physiologists, Gibson and Cooke, realized the need for a standard technique for collecting sweat for testing, and described a method of stimulating sweat production and collecting it.

One of the symptoms considered as an almost certain sign of CF was, in fact, first described in 1905 by Landsteiner. In translation, the title of his article reads: 'Intestinal obstruction from thickened meconium'. The first dark-green stools passed after birth are called meconium, and meconium ileus (an obstruction of the small intestine) affects 10–15 per cent of those infants destined to show the other signs of CF.

Poor absorption of food is a characteristic of most people with CF who go untreated. It manifests itself as steatorrhoea (non-digestion of fat leading to bulky, strong-smelling stools). There are also a number of other ways in which the disease may show its presence. In infants, the steatorrhoea may be accompanied by prolapse of the rectum (a condition where the very frequent passage of bulky stools causes the lining of the rectum to protrude through the anus). The first symptoms of CF in the young child are often confused with milk allergy.

Cystic fibrosis sufferers are also subject to recurrent chest infections. These are caused by bacteria, notably *Staphylococcus aureus* and the different types of *Pseudomonas*. While the former is an aggressive bacterium that causes disease in healthy people, the latter is an opportunist, that requires a weakness in the tissue it is attacking before it can gain a foothold. Conditions in the lungs of CF patients provide the right environment for both organisms to thrive and generally, although not always, one or other organism is found. Before anti-staphylococcal antibiotics were discovered, *Staphylococcus aureus* predominated. The effects of repeated chest infections usually led to death by seven years of age. Now, survival is much longer and a progression from staphylococcal to pseudomonal infection is common in those patients more severely affected.

As suggested above, there is great variation in the severity of CF, even within members of the same family. A number of studies have shown that girls with CF generally do slightly worse than boys. Nevertheless, a good number of affected girls have grown up to have children. The vast majority of men with CF are sterile; Shwachman showed in 1968 that this was due to fibrosis of the epididymis and absence of a vas deferens. These two ducts normally form a conduit through which sperm pass on their way from the testis to the exterior of the body.

Puberty may be delayed in CF sufferers, especially if they are underweight and undersized for their age. These symptoms can result in psychological problems in adolescence. The child may question treatment at this stage and normal adolescent rebellion can result in the breaking of dietary restrictions and resistance to physiotherapy and taking medicines.

Cystic fibrosis is a hereditary disease. Cedric Carter, in 1952, was the first to recognize the way in which the CF gene is transmitted from one generation to the next. The disease is caused by a pair of abnormal *recessive* genes in each cell of the body (a gene is a small portion of the genetic material, that is concerned with the making of a protein). The effects of a single recessive gene are masked when the normal form of the same gene also occurs in the same cell in a carrier. The defective gene in CF is on an autosome, the disease occurring equally often in males and females (this is discussed further in Chapter 6). The illness CF affects only those individuals who have inherited the defective gene from *both* their mother and father. If two carriers marry there is a one in four chance that any of their offspring may inherit the gene from each of them. No adverse health problems occur for the parents through being carriers.

Cystic fibrosis is the commonest autosomal recessive genetic disease of white Indo-Europeans (Caucasians). In most parts of the world, between 1 in 1500 and 1 in 2500 Caucasian children are born with CF, though the disease may not be apparent at birth. If one takes these two sets of figures and assumes that all CF arises from the same gene, then between 1 in 16 and 1 in 25 Caucasians is a carrier.

On average, one child with CF is born every day in the United Kingdom, and four to five daily in the United States. In fact, the condition occurs wherever Europeans have settled. It is extremely rare in the Chinese, and in the Negro races in Africa. In some Third World countries, with high infant mortality, a diagnosis of CF could easily be missed. In Britain, we do see CF in children of Pakistani and Arab descent. The incidence in their countries of origin is unknown.

Until recently there was no reliable test to detect a CF carrier, and carrier status could only be established after the birth of a CF child to a particular couple. Over the last couple of years, research advances have dramatically altered this situation. In many cases we can now tell if a person drawn at random from the general population carries a CF gene, by directly testing his or her genetic material. In other words, that person does not have to produce a CF child before we know that he or she carries a CF gene. Precisely how this test is done will be explained more fully in Chapter 6. It is likely that in the next few years it will become possible to test the majority of the population, should they wish it, to see who carries a CF gene.

Late in 1985, it was established by research groups in Denmark, Canada, America, and England that the gene causing CF was located on chromosome 7. Nearly four years later, in September 1989, a tremendous research effort from several large groups of scientists culminated in the publication, in the American journal *Science*, of the isolation of the CF gene itself. Collaborating research groups in Canada and North America had finally achieved the feat that the CF world had been awaiting for so long. However, it should be remembered that this is really only the beginning of the story in terms of understanding how the CF gene acts to cause the disease. In the piece of genetic information that is the

CF gene, research scientists now have the tool to start asking funda-mental questions about the disease process in CF and how more effective treatments might be developed.

Despite the lack of information on the basic defect, an aggressive approach to treatment has resulted in increased survival and improved health for CF sufferers. Time out of school or off work has been reduced through better attention to chest infections, a positive attitude to chest physiotherapy, adequate dietary intake, and early recognition of danger signs. Treatment is best co-ordinated in a multidisciplinary CF clinic and is mostly on an out-patient basis. Certain treatments have not stood the test of time. Notable among these is the use of mist tents, in which affected children used to sleep, and special low fat diets. We continue to search for effective treatments and to question the necessity of treat-ments that involve sacrifice of time or convenience by the affected person. Unfortunately, many of the effective treatments do require such sacrifice.

There is controversy about many aspects of CF treatment. In the long term, it is hoped that the discovery of the CF gene will enable aspects of treatment to become simpler, more directly aimed at correcting the basic defect in the disease and so less controversial. In writing a book on 'the facts' we have tried hard to be objective and to highlight the more readily acceptable points.

2

What is happening in the body in cystic fibrosis?

Three main systems in the body are classically affected by cystic fibrosis. These are the lungs and respiratory tract, the digestive system (particularly the pancreas and intestines) and the sweat glands. In this chapter the effects of CF on each of these three systems will be discussed in more detail.

THE LUNGS AND RESPIRATORY TRACT

Figure 1 shows the normal anatomy of the respiratory tree. Air enters through the nostrils into the nasal sinuses, then passes into the single tube of the trachea or windpipe. The trachea splits at its bottom end into two bronchi (one for each lung), and the bronchi continue to divide into smaller and smaller tubes (bronchioles), ending in thousands of small air sacs or alveoli. It is from the alveoli that oxygen enters the bloodstream and carbon dioxide is released.

From the upper airways down to the bronchioles, the respiratory tree is lined with many small, hair-like protrusions called cilia. The cilia are covered in a thin layer of mucus. They beat in a wave-like motion to waft the mucus and any extraneous matter (including bacteria) towards the nose or pharynx. Whatever reaches the upper part of the respiratory tree is either swallowed or coughed out. Ciliary action will normally act against gravity to clear the various lobes of the lung, whatever position the body may be in.

In CF, however, mucus tends to clog up the upper and lower respiratory tree. The reasons for this are not clear. It is possible that as a secondary effect of the basic defect in CF the mucous secretions contain less water than they should, though this is a controversial suggestion. It is clear from detailed research that poor mucus clearance is not due to uneven ciliary beating (the synchronized beating of cilia lining the respiratory tree normally wafts mucus upwards and out of the lungs).

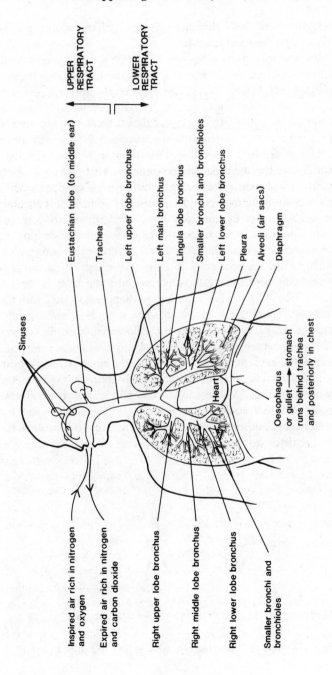

Fig. 1. Diagram of a transverse section through the human respiratory tree.

However, there is no doubt that mucus is poorly cleared against gravity in the presence of bacterial infection.

Build-up of mucus in the lungs can have several consequences. Ball-valve effects occur in those segments of the lung that have become overdistended because air passes an obstruction on breathing in, but does not all pass back on breathing out. These obstructions are caused by mucus and airway narrowing. The overinflation becomes more marked with time, and results in emphysema, a state of overdistension in which the elasticity of the lung is reduced. Deformity of the chest develops, with rounding of the shoulders and prominence of the sternum. Occasionally, and usually late in the course of the disease, distended alveoli at the surface of the lung may rupture, giving rise to pneumothorax (air between the surface of the lung and the chest wall) requiring special treatment. This damage is compounded by recurrent or continuous chest infections, or by bronchiectasis, a state of permanent weakening of the bronchial walls and poor drainage of infected mucus. Bronchiectasis is associated with permanent lung infection and clubbing of the fingers (see Fig. 2). Clubbing occurs as a result of substances associated with the lung infections entering the blood. In some way these stimulate the growth of the soft tissue at the bases of the finger and toenails, causing loss of the angle between the nail and the skin.

Abnormalities in the air and blood supply to the lungs may result from CF. These abnormalities may not be immediately apparent, as the reserve capacity of the lungs allows them to function normally even when quite significantly damaged. Studies with radioactive compounds either injected into a vein or inhaled (see Chapter 3, p. 41, and Fig. 10) can show the extent of the tissue damage.

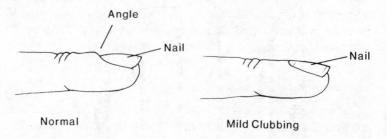

Fig. 2. Diagram of finger clubbing (see also Key to Fig. 9, p. 34).

Bacterial infections in the respiratory tree in CF

Though a number of bacterial chest infections may occur in CF, the commonest is caused by *Staphylococcus aureus*. Later in the course of the disease, infection by *Pseudomonas* bacteria may also occur. *Staphylococcus aureus* is a micro-organism that does not occur in the body naturally, but only as part of an infection. It may cause minor problems such as pimples, or more major ones like osteomyelitis (a bone infection) in the general population, but in CF it is found together with chronic (long-term) bronchitis and lung infection. The bacterium *Pseudomonas aeruginosa* does not infect healthy tissue. It only attacks damaged tissue, for example the skin in severe burns, or the lungs in CF, when a certain degree of damage and loss of some of the healthy lining of the bronchi has occurred. Different varieties of *Pseudomonas* are recognized by their laboratory characteristics (see Fig. 3). There seem to be two forms of the bacteria, non-mucoid and mucoid. The mucoid type has a slimy appearance and once acquired it is seldom eradicated. Though a cause of less tissue damage than *Staphylococcus*, an established mucoid *Pseudomonas* infection is generally associated with deterioration in lung function.

The upper respiratory tract in CF

Cystic fibrosis may cause changes in the nose and in other parts of the respiratory tree above the trachea. Nasal polyps (protruberant growths of the mucous membranes) develop in the nose in many older children. They occasionally require surgical removal, but have a tendency to recur.

THE GASTRO-INTESTINAL TRACT

The effects of CF on the gastro-intestinal tract are numerous and complex. To help understand them more fully, an outline of the normal processes of digestion and metabolism of food is given below.

Introduction to digestion and metabolism

In the normal digestive process, food is broken down both mechanically (chewing) and chemically from complex molecules such as proteins, fats, and carbohydrates (starch) to smaller, simpler molecules such as amino acids, fatty acids and sugars. This allows the food to be absorbed into the

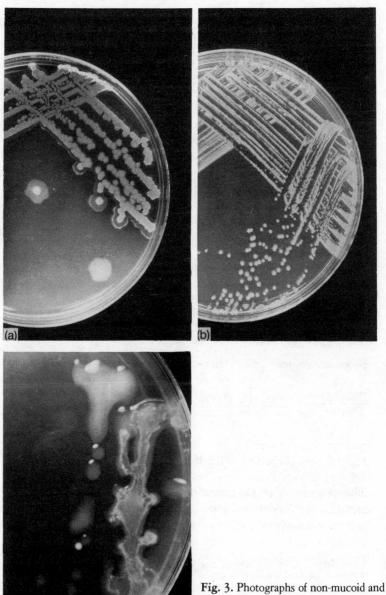

Fig. 3. Photographs of non-mucoid and mucoid *Pseudomonas* colonies on Agar culture plates. (a) non-mucoid, rough; (b) non-mucoid, smooth; (c) mucoid.

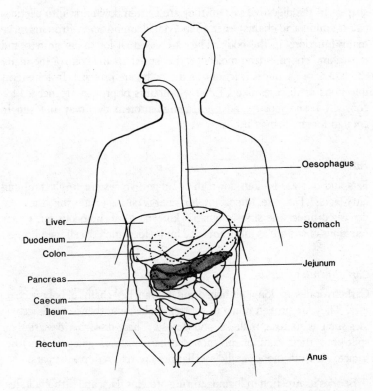

Oesophagus

Liver

Duodenum

Colon

Pancreas

Caecum

Ileum

Rectum

Stomach

Jejunum

Anus

Fig. 4. Diagram of a transverse section through the human digestive system.

body through the walls of the small intestine or ileum (see Fig. 4), and then transported in the blood to the liver. The liver is the central chemical factory of the body: here the amino acids and other small molecules are used as building blocks for the body's own proteins, carbohydrates, etc. These then circulate in the bloodstream and are taken up by the various body tissues (e.g. lungs, muscles, brain etc.) as they need them. Tissues need a constant supply of proteins and other nutrients because many cells live only a few days or weeks and there is a constant replacement of dead or dying cells.

Let us look briefly at the individual food types and their fates.

Proteins

Proteins are made of long chains of amino acids, coiled into complex shapes. In the digestive system they are broken down first into peptides (short amino acid chains), then to individual amino acids. Proteins serve many functions in the body. They are essential for tissue growth and repair, and enzymes (the molecules that speed up and control the many thousands of chemical reactions in the body) are proteins. In long-term infections or diseases like CF, large amounts of protein are needed for constant tissue repair, and even a high protein diet may not supply enough for the body's needs.

Fats

Fats and oils are broken down in the digestive system to glycerol and fatty acids. Fats are important for energy storage: for this they are deposited under the skin in what is known as subcutaneous fat. Other functions of fats are as lubricants and in the formation of cell membranes.

Carbohydrates (starch)

Carbohydrates are long, branched and unbranched chains of polysaccharides. They are broken down to shorter chains, and thence to disaccharides such as sucrose, maltose, and lactose. These disaccharides are then split into their component monosaccharides (e.g. glucose, fructose, galactose). Both mono- and disaccharides are referred to as sugars.

Besides its function in manufacturing proteins, fats, and carbohydrates, the liver is responsible for the breakdown and detoxification of waste products in the body. These waste products then pass out of the body in the urine or faeces. The body uses only glucose products in metabolism and so, in the liver, all monosaccharides are converted to glucose compounds. Glucose is the main fuel for the chemical cycle that supplies energy for the body's functions. Ready glucose energy is stored in the liver and muscles as glycogen. When glycogen stores are full, the excess is stored as fat.

The digestive tract

The parts of the digestive tract (see Fig. 4) involved in each step of digestion are as follows. In the mouth food particles are reduced in size by the teeth and the digestion of starch begins with the action of the enzyme amylase present in saliva. The smell and taste of food stimulate the production of saliva and also of gastrin, a hormone (see Glossary for definition) which acts on the stomach to stimulate the production of enzymes there. After being swallowed, food travels down the oesophagus or gullet to the stomach. (Transport of food through the digestive tract is achieved by the action of muscles in the gut wall.) Food stays in the stomach for about four hours, during which time it mixes with hydrochloric acid and the enzyme pepsin (pepsin is responsible for breaking down the protein in the diet to peptides). The food is prevented from leaving the stomach by a valve called the pylorus, which closes off the entrance to the duodenum. The presence of food in the stomach stimulates the production of a hormone called secretin. This hormone travels in the bloodstream to the duodenum, the liver, and the pancreas, where it stimulates the production of digestive juices.

After four hours in the stomach the food is in the form of a ball or bolus. The pyloric valve then opens, and this bolus of food passes into the duodenum. There it encounters an alkaline digestive fluid consisting of bicarbonate, bile, and the enzymes trypsin, amylase, and lipase from the pancreas. Trypsin completes the breaking down of peptides to amino acids. Amylase continues with the breaking down of starch to the disaccharides sucrose, maltose, and lactose. Further enzymes from the walls of the duodenum itself break down the disaccharides to their component monosaccharides. Fats are emulsified by the bile and then broken down by lipase to glycerol and fatty acids.

From the duodenum, the food travels slowly down through the jejunum and ileum. This whole section of the digestive tract is lined with tiny villi, folds in the gut lining, that increase the surface area available for food absorption. Amino acids, monosaccharides, and the smaller fat breakdown products are absorbed into the blood vessels lining the villi and transported from there to the liver. Larger fat breakdown products enter the lymph channels or lacteals. (The lymphatic system, like the blood system, transports materials around the body and helps to defend it from infection.) In the lymph channels the fat particles are coated, rendering them more soluble, before they enter the bloodstream and eventually reach the liver.

Certain substances in the diet that cannot be digested act as roughage, helping to increase the bulk of the bolus and help its passage down the intestinal canal. Notable amongst these is a polysaccharide, raffinose, which forms the fibres in many vegetables. The process of digestion continues all the way down to the end of the ileum.

At the end of the ileum, undigested material passes into the caecum, a mixing chamber. From there it enters the colon where much of the water is reabsorbed. Bacteria normally present in the caecum and colon act on the waste products to break them down into faeces by a process of fermentation. The fermentation also results in the formation of gas (flatus or wind). If there is poor absorption of food, especially of fat, this process of fermentation is especially active, and faeces and flatus become foul-smelling. This happens in a person with CF either taking a diet too rich in fat or receiving too little pancreatic supplement. Carbohydrates can also ferment in the intestine, though special forms of carbohydrate such as Polycal® and Hical® are less subject to fermentation. These compounds can be used in CF to increase energy intake without unpleasant side-effects.

The pancreas and CF

As has already been mentioned, one of the major effects of cystic fibrosis is on the pancreas. Replacement of pancreatic cells with fibrous scar tissue begins before birth, and generally gets worse with time. As a result of this tissue damage, caused initially by deposits of dried up secretions, the pancreas ceases to function properly. Production of pancreatic juices decreases, and as we saw previously this juice contains enzymes essential for the breakdown and absorption of food. In this section we will look in more detail at the function of the pancreas and how it is affected by CF.

The pancreas secretes mainly water, bicarbonate, and protein enzymes. Secretion of pancreatic juices is a continuous process, but the presence of food in the stomach, or certain other stimuli, can increase the rate of secretion. Bicarbonate secreted in the pancreatic juice is essential in changing the pH of the duodenal contents from the acidic stomach pH to the alkaline pH at which pancreatic enzymes function best. (pH is a measure of acidity or alkalinity.) There is some evidence that there is reduced bicarbonate secretion in CF pancreatic juices.

Pancreatic enzymes are responsible for the breakdown of many components of the diet. Brief descriptions of the actions of the three major pancreatic enzymes were given in the previous section. After absorption and entry into the bloodstream these building blocks provide the essential substances for body growth and repair and the fuels on which the body functions.

Malabsorption

As described earlier, when foodstuffs are not adequately digested they cannot be absorbed normally from the intestines. This results in a wide range of symptoms due to abnormal excretion of fat in the faeces (steatorrhoea) and deficiency of vitamins soluble in fat, as well as proteins, minerals, carbohydrates, other vitamins, and water. Steatorrhoea is a major problem in inadequately treated CF. Furthermore, because the fat is only partly digested, it causes irritation of the bowel and this in turn leads to an increase in the frequency and rate of passage of bowel contents.

Deficiency of the enzyme trypsin means that some of the protein in the diet is not fully broken down to amino acids in the duodenum. Some peptide fragments remain, and since these cannot be absorbed, they pass into the lower intestine and bowel. Here they are broken down to amino acids by other enzymes and by bacteria. As a result, large amounts of amino acids find their way into the faeces, where together with undigested fat they produce a pronounced odour.

The obvious treatment for malabsorption of food is to try and supplement the levels of natural digestive enzymes. Simultaneously, factors that are lacking from the diet due to abnormal digestion and absorption must be introduced into the body by some other route in order to prevent malnutrition. These therapeutic approaches are dealt with in more detail in Chapter 3. Since pancreatic enzymes do not reach the intestine in most cases of CF, pancreatic enzyme supplements are an essential part of treatment. A small percentage of CF patients have normal pancreatic function.

Gastro-intestinal symptoms of CF

During the newborn period: meconium ileus

The first stools of a newborn baby are called meconium. Ten to fifteen per cent of the babies with CF have intestinal obstruction in the first few days of life. The small intestine is clogged with sticky meconium, presumably because of thickened mucus from the intestinal glands. This blockage of the lower intestine causes bilious vomiting and swelling of the abdomen. X-rays help to distinguish meconium ileus from other causes of intestinal blockage.

Surgery is generally necessary in meconium ileus, though the administration of hygroscopic (water-attracting) enemas or the use of other substances capable of thinning mucus may occasionally be effective. The most successful operation has been Bishop and Koop's ileostomy. This entails bringing a loop of the ileum to open on the abdominal wall. Stools

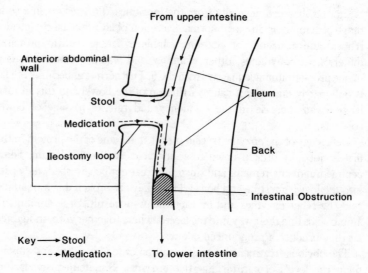

Fig. 5. Diagram of Bishop–Koop ileostomy.

can then be passed above the blockage, while medication can be given through the opening to clear the obstruction (see Fig. 5). Once the lower bowel has been unblocked, stools can once again pass along the normal channel and the ileostomy can be closed. This generally takes between one and three months to happen. The immediate prognosis (i.e. chances of recovery from) of meconium ileus improved markedly after introduction of the ileostomy operation in the late 1960s.

Care of newborn babies before and after operations has improved greatly in the last ten years. As a result, it has become possible for some infants with meconium ileus to have a much simpler operation. In the new operation the most obstructed part of the bowel is simply removed, and the two cut ends are joined.

It is a myth to suppose that children born with meconium ileus and thus diagnosed as having CF at birth are less prone to lung disease. While meconium ileus almost always implies the presence of CF in Caucasians, this is not invariable. Confirmation of CF by the sweat test is very important in any case of meconium ileus.

The most serious complication of meconium ileus is meconium peritonitis, an acute inflammation of the membrane that lines the abdomen (the peritoneum). Meconium peritonitis may be present at birth. It occurs when a hole develops in the wall of a section of bowel blocked by meconium. The meconium spills into the peritoneum and causes inflammation.

Attacks of incomplete intestinal obstruction may occasionally occur later in life from build-up of faeces and mucus. These have been labelled meconium ileus equivalent, but they bear no relationship to the condition affecting the newborn (see later in this section).

There is good evidence of a tendency for meconium ileus to recur within families. If meconium ileus is found in one member of a family, there is a 50 per cent chance of it occurring in other CF children in the same family.

Meconium ileus or meconium peritonitis may affect the unborn child and may occasionally result in spontaneous late miscarriage, stillbirth, or premature birth.

After the newborn period

Symptoms of gastro-intestinal abnormalities in CF are often seen before symptoms in the respiratory system or elsewhere. The most pronounced symptom is steatorrhoea, fatty or loose, strong-smelling stools. It is often associated with abdominal distension. Steatorrhoea is the indirect result of the fibrous scarring of the pancreas from which CF derives its name. The fibrous tissue blocks the ducts of the pancreas and eventually stops the pancreatic digestive juices from reaching the small intestine to digest the food. This process, which is already well established by birth, in turn causes nutrients to be inefficiently absorbed. It is poor digestion of fat, particularly, that gives the faeces in steatorrhoea their characteristic look, hence the name steatorrhoea (*steato* being the Greek word for fat, and *rhoia* for flowing). Certain amino acids do not depend on the pancreas for breakdown but are nevertheless poorly absorbed, showing that the small intestine itself is not functioning perfectly in CF.

Rectal prolapse. In this condition, malabsorption of fat, with very frequent stools, results in the inner lining of the rectum protruding through the anus. CF should be considered in any infant with a prolapsed rectum. Rectal prolapse should come under ready control if dietary fat is reduced and pancreatic enzymes are given with the feeds.

Meconium ileus equivalent. This rather poor term is used for attacks of complete or partial intestinal obstruction that may occur later on in the life of a person with CF. Attacks occur mainly as a result of blockage caused by mucus and fatty stools. In some CF adults abdominal pain and attacks of such obstruction may be the main complaint. The condition is not more common amongst those who had meconium ileus at birth. Recent improvements in the treatment of CF have reduced the incidence of this complication.

Intussusception.   In this disorder a portion of small intestine closer to the stomach folds into the adjoining region of the downstream bowel, threatening the blood supply of the trapped inner portion (see Fig. 6). Intussusception is a rare but potentially serious complication of CF. Treatment is nearly always by operation.

The liver and biliary tree

Cirrhosis (fibrous scarring) of the liver occurs in about 5 per cent of people with CF. In this disorder, the fibrous tissue laid down partially blocks the veins draining into the liver from the intestine and spleen. As the fibrous tissue contracts (part of the natural progression of any fibrotic process), the liver cells may be damaged. As a result they are unable to carry out their normal tasks. The partial blockage of the blood supply to the spleen causes it to enlarge, and the veins at the lower end of the

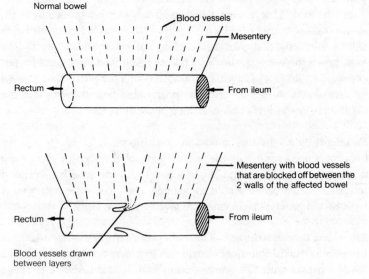

Fig. 6. Diagram of intussusception.

oesophagus may also become swollen and varicosed. These varices (or dilated veins) may bleed on occasion and require the injection of sclerosing agents, which strengthen the blood vessel wall. Though this is a potentially serious complication that can cause jaundice, liver failure, and bleeding, in CF it is more common to see mild cases, which run a course over many years. Even after a more serious manifestation, the condition may improve. Why only a few CF patients have this complication is not fully understood. It is not necessarily the older or the more severely ill who are affected in this way. The newborn with CF may sometimes show prolonged jaundice, possibly because of mucus in the bile channels. This resolves with time and is not especially associated with liver disease later in life.

Diabetes

Most children with diabetes have so-called insulin-dependent diabetes. Two hormones, insulin and glucagon, are produced by the pancreas, in groups of cells known as the Islets of Langerhans. Glucagon is produced by alpha cells in these regions, while insulin is produced by beta cells. Insulin lowers the levels of sugar (glucose) in the blood by converting it to the carbohydrate glycogen, which is stored in the liver. Glucagon is one of the hormones that reconverts glycogen to glucose.

In insulin-dependent diabetes most of the beta cells (those manufacturing insulin) are destroyed. However, diabetes in people with CF is caused by contraction of fibrous scar tissue, which destroys limited numbers of both alpha and beta cells. The resulting diabetes, which may first appear in the early teens, is generally mild and easily controlled with small doses of insulin. The more severe complications of diabetes such as coma and acidosis (a build up of acids in the blood) are unusual. Long-term kidney complications do not occur. About 3 per cent of adolescents and adults with CF develop diabetes.

Rare gastro-intestinal manifestations in CF

Oedema is a generalized body swelling caused by low levels of the protein albumin in the blood. Albumin is involved in the process of keeping fluid in the blood vessels. When albumin is deficient, fluid builds up in the tissues. Oedema is sometimes found as a sign of cystic fibrosis in young infants. On occasion this has happened when the first loose stools have been misdiagnosed as milk allergy and soya feeds have been given.

Absence of gastro-intestinal symptoms

A small proportion of people with CF have no problems with their digestive system. This lack of symptoms is difficult to understand. Some studies claim that as many as 10 per cent of CF patients show no gastro-intestinal problems. The diagnosis of CF may be suspect in some of this 10 per cent. On the other hand, if one only suspects CF when there *are* gastro-intestinal symptoms, one may underdiagnose this category of patients. There is undoubtedly a well-described group of pancreatic sufficient CF patients, in other words, CFs who have a pancreas that functions normally or close to normal. It seems likely from genetic data that this group of patients may have a different defect in the same gene. That is, the majority of CFs who have pancreatic insufficiency have a genetic alteration that has more pronounced effects on the functioning of the cystic fibrosis gene product.

THE SWEAT GLAND

Sweat consists of a weak solution of electrolytes (electrically charged molecules) in water. These are mainly sodium and chloride, with some calcium and some potassium. The electrolyte solution has the same pH as the blood, being slightly alkaline. In CF there is a marked increase of these electrolytes in the sweat, because the reabsorption of chloride is impaired. The reason for this impaired absorption has not yet been established. It is known that the basic defect in CF is expressed as an abnormal regulation of the movements of salt across the layer of cells that line certain specialized ducts such as the sweat gland duct. Unlike other organs affected by CF, the sweat gland and its duct appear normal when examined under the microscope.

THE REPRODUCTIVE SYSTEM

One of the most consistent findings in men with CF is an abnormality of the epididymis and vas deferens (the tubes that carry sperm from the testes (see Fig. 7)). These tubes end in blind channels instead of connecting through to the urethra. In fact, the epididymis is usually blocked and the vas deferens may be completely absent. During fetal life, the male genital duct system appears intact in CF. It seems likely that sometime

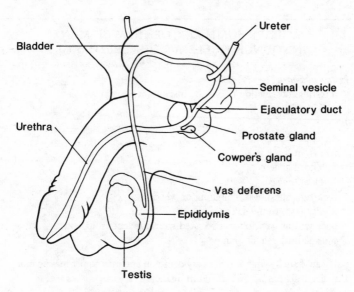

Fig. 7. Diagram of the male reproductive system.

before birth the duct system becomes blocked by mucous secretions as occurs in the pancreatic duct in CF. This blockage may then result in gradual destruction of the vas deferens. At least 97 per cent of males with CF are affected in this way from birth. As a result, most men with CF are sterile, although there have been documented cases of men with CF producing normal sperm and, in a few instances, of fathering children.

There are no equivalent changes in the female reproductive tract, and increasing numbers of women with CF are giving birth to children. In several reported instances the children born also had CF. (Of course, all children born to a woman with CF must of necessity be carriers of the disease; see Chapter 6.) Occasionally, reduced amounts of the mucus that normally lubricates the female reproductive tract cause infertility in women with CF.

A BRIEF SUMMARY OF HOW CF MAY ANNOUNCE ITSELF AT DIFFERENT AGES

In the newborn:
  intestinal obstruction caused by meconium ileus or atresia;
  prolonged jaundice.
Infants:
  rectal prolapse;
  recurrent loose stools;
  distended abdomen;
  'milk allergy';
  recurrent chestiness, coughing or wheezing;
  a salty taste to the sweat;
  poor weight gain, often associated with a ravenous appetite;
  unexplained dehydration.

Because such symptoms are very common and may sometimes be mild, the diagnosis can be overlooked in infancy.
In older children:
  after the diagnosis of CF in a brother or sister;
  incomplete intestinal obstruction;
  nasal polyps, especially if recurrent;
  bronchiectasis or recurrent chest infections;
  heat prostration;
  underweight child.

Occasionally the diagnosis may be missed for many years.
In adolescents or adults:
  delayed onset of puberty;
  sterile or azospermic males;
  infertile females with scanty cervical mucus.
  bronchiectasis

HOW IS A DIAGNOSIS OF CF CONFIRMED?

In most circumstances, CF can be confirmed in children by a carefully performed sweat test. In the sweat test, a small amount of pilocarpine (a sweating promoter) is driven into the skin by stimulation with a few amperes of electric current (this process is known as iontophoresis). When the sweating rate is adequate, the concentrations of sodium and chloride (i.e. salt) in the sweat are measured.

In a normal child the sweat will contain sodium and chloride in concentrations of between fifteen and thirty millimoles per litre (mmol l^{-1}). Concentrations of sodium and chloride greater than 70 mmol l^{-1} are diagnostic of CF. This means that children with CF have two to five times the normal amount of salt in their sweat. A concentration of sodium and chloride well above 70 mmol l^{-1} does not indicate that the disease will be more severe.

The sweat test is quite safe and very reliable, but it needs to be performed by experienced staff. Stimulation of an adequate sweating rate in very young infants can sometimes be a problem. The recent introduction of a system that employs capillary pressure to suck up sweat into polythene tubing has made sweat testing easier and more efficient.

The sweat test is the least unpleasant method of diagnosis. In cases where the results of this test are borderline, it may be necessary to measure the pancreatic secretions directly, and check whether these secretions are reaching the duodenum. For this test it used to be necessary to insert a small tube into the duodenum via the mouth, but the test can now be done more simply by taking a urine sample and measuring substances in the urine that depend on pancreatic function.

It should be noted that in people with CF who have no intestinal troubles (see earlier section), the pancreatic secretion results would be near normal.

Occasionally, CF may go undiagnosed for many years, in which case it could be necessary to recognize the disease in an adult. For adults, the normal range of salt concentration in sweat is greater than for children, and the sweat test rather loses its value in diagnosis. Men thought to have CF can be tested for azospermia (absence of sperm in the ejaculate). Since the discovery of the actual gene defect (see chapter 6) a diagnosis of CF can now be made in about two thirds of cases by DNA analysis.

SHOULD WE SCREEN THE NEWBORN FOR CF?

The validity of testing all newborn babies for CF is still a matter of debate. A simple test (BM Meconium) exists, which works on the principle that the albumin content of the meconium is increased in newborns with CF. This has been used in some countries over the past decade. A more reliable test is the measurement of serum immune-reactive trypsin (IRT) in a specimen of blood. This test is based on the observed reaction of the body's antibody defences to the pancreatic enzyme trypsin. A raised level of the antibody is found in the blood of most newborns with CF.

Following the recent isolation of the CF gene it will soon be possible to detect CF by a simple test carried out on the genetic material of the majority of babies at birth. All that will be required will be a very small blood-sample, such as that currently taken routinely as a 'heel prick' from all new born babies to test for another inherited disorder called PKU (phenylketonuria). At present (Spring 1990) such a test of the genetic material could only detect about 70 per cent of CFs in the UK and possibly rather less than this in southern European populations. It is likely that before long nearly all CF individuals will be identifiable by this method.

Advantages and problems of screening

There have been significant problems with the BM meconium and IRT screening tests, mainly due to their lack of reliability in some screening laboratories. In other words, some normal babies were diagnosed as having CF and some CF babies were not detected. However, the new tests, that will analyse the genetic material directly for the presence of cystic fibrosis genes, should be almost one hundred per cent reliable. This will rather change the balance of the CF screening debate. In the UK, the availability of a CF test is likely to depend on the willingness or ability of regional health authorities to pay for this service. Where private health care predominates, the cost of a perinatal CF test will undoubtedly also be important.

The most controversial question relating to newborn screening for CF is whether the eventual prognosis is altered by early diagnosis. This remains extraordinarily difficult to prove. Unfortunately, the strongest argument for screening remains the ease with which a diagnosis of CF may be overlooked, some children having had symptoms for a long time before the diagnosis of CF is considered or made. In one study, the *average* delay between onset of symptoms (excluding meconium ileus) and diagnosis was 13 months. This delay can cause psychological problems—parents may feel guilty about not noticing ill effects earlier, or may blame the general practitioner for not recognizing the symptoms when he first saw the child.

By allowing very early diagnosis, screening would sometimes prevent the birth of a second affected child.

When a truly effective early treatment for CF becomes available, capable of greatly reducing damage to the pancreas and lungs, then the case for screening will be made. Until then, it is important that paediatricians educate themselves, general practitioners, and the public about the early signs of CF.

3

Treatment of cystic fibrosis

THE CF CLINIC—A MULTIDISCIPLINARY APPROACH

Treatment of CF in a special clinic allows a local body of expertise to build up, to help manage the many complex ways in which the illness can affect a person. Greater longevity and improved health have been directly ascribed to special clinic treatment as opposed to care of the child by the paediatrician or medical practitioner alone.

An efficient CF clinic has a team of trained staff. The team is led by a paediatrician and consists of a nursing sister, who works exclusively with CF patients (she has home and hospital contact with the families); a physiotherapist interested in sports medicine and lung function; a dietician; a psychologist; and a social worker. The parents are the most important members of the treatment team, and later the child him/herself. Continuity is the greatest secret of success. At the clinic at the Royal Manchester Children's Hospital (RMCH), the nursing assistant who helps at the clinic has been attached to it for 10 years and knows all sorts of family details which have proved important from time to time. We believe patients can be better treated at a special CF clinic than at a respiratory or gastro-intestinal clinic that includes patients with CF. Unless there are insuperable geographical problems, a CF clinic should probably have a minimum of 10 patients and a maximum of 40 to each paediatrician. A working party of the British Paediatric Association recommended that each affected person should be known to a major CF clinic, with care shared between this clinic, paediatricians, physicians, and local general practitioners.

Many children with CF live some way away from the CF centre. Shared care between the clinic and the local paediatrician is becoming popular. One American study showed that the long-term outlook for CF patients was closely related to the frequency with which they were seen by health professionals. Obviously, shared care increases the efficiency of disease surveillance.

With improved survival, more 'adult' CF clinics are coming into being. The age at which patients move to the adult clinic varies according to local facilities and expertise, but it may be as early as 16 years old. In some centres the physician and paediatrician run joint clinics and achieve continuity that way.

At the RMCH the 80 patients we have at present attend the weekly clinic by appointment where possible, though at any other time an open door policy operates to clinic attendance and to the in-patients ward. The patient and parents will see the paediatrician on each visit to the clinic, and often see other members of the team informally in the large ante-room containing the scales and lung-function equipment. Team members might check on aspects of dietary care, or the efficiency of the parents' physiotherapy techniques in this way. Of course if a specific problem arises requiring detailed involvement of one of the team members (for example the psychologist), special arrangements can be made.

On a normal visit to the clinic, a patient is weighed, their height is recorded, and various measurements of lung function are taken. An instrument called a spirometer is used to measure lung function. The patient breathes into this apparatus, which measures the air capacity of the lungs, plus the speed and volume of air moved in and out of the lungs in breathing (see Fig. 8).

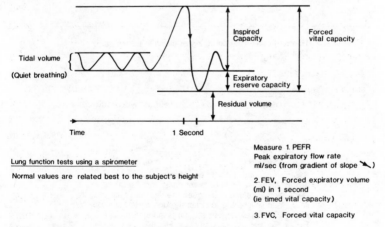

Fig. 8. Diagram to show the theory of lung function tests:

Key: Forced vital capacity = total volume of air that can be moved.
Inspired capacity = volume of air taken into the lungs on breathing in.
Expiratory reserve capacity = the extra volume of air which can be breathed out at the end of quiet expiration.
Residual volume = the air which remains in the lung after deepest expiration.

The findings of the physical examination are recorded on a proforma (Fig. 9), along with information on the patient's lung and bowel condition, their school or work attendance, and their treatment. The proforma shown in Fig. 9 is the one used at RMCH. We are encouraging neighbouring clinics in our region to use the same proforma so that computer comparisons can be made between subjects at different clinics.

After each clinic session, a round-table discussion of those people seen at the clinic or in the ward takes place between all the staff members. Aspects of management and any planned or on-going research are discussed in practical terms at this meeting. Patients are seen a minimum of once every three months at the RMCH clinic, but many have more frequent contact through home visits from the CF Nursing Sister.

The hospital-based social worker has close contacts with many families and is especially involved with one-parent families and those with pressing financial or domestic problems. While she helps the families over various difficulties she has the opportunity of getting to know them well and to ensure that contacts with the clinic are maintained and attendance is regular. She acts on the families' behalf in processing claims for attendance allowance. From her training she complements the work of the clinical psychologist and clinic nurse.

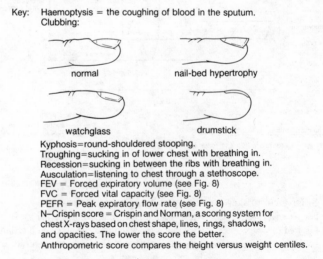

Key: Haemoptysis = the coughing of blood in the sputum.
Clubbing:

normal   nail-bed hypertrophy

watchglass   drumstick

Kyphosis=round-shouldered stooping.
Troughing=sucking in of lower chest with breathing in.
Recession=sucking in between the ribs with breathing in.
Ausculation=listening to chest through a stethoscope.
FEV = Forced expiratory volume (see Fig. 8)
FVC = Forced vital capacity (see Fig. 8)
PEFR = Peak expiratory flow rate (see Fig. 8)
N–Crispin score = Crispin and Norman, a scoring system for chest X-rays based on chest shape, lines, rings, shadows, and opacities. The lower the score the better.
Anthropometric score compares the height versus weight centiles.

Fig. 9. A CF clinic recording chart or proforma. (From the Royal Manchester Children's Hospital Cystic Fibrosis Clinic.)

ROYAL MANCHESTER CHILDREN'S HOSPITAL
CYSTIC FIBROSIS CLINIC

Date...../..../....   Name...   Age...............YRS.

General Comments

....

....

....

....

Exercise Intol, ☐   0. None   1. Slight   2. Severe

Cough ☐   0. None   1. After Physio   2. Occasional   3. Daily

Wheeze ☐   0. None   1. Occasional   2. Regular

Sputum ☐   0. None   1. After Physio   2. Little   3. Lot
Haemoptysis ☐   y/n

Appetite ☐   0. Normal   1. Reduced   2. Increased

No of Stools ☐   Per day

Stool consistency ☐   0. Normal   1. Loose   2. Bulky

Smelly stools ☐   y/n

Abdominal Pain ☐   y/n

Immunizations   Pertussis ☐
Measles ☐
Influenza ☐

0. No immunization yet-needs it
1. Has had first dose
2. Has had second dose
3. Completed course
4. Immunization not essential
5. Immunization contraindicated

Physio frequency ☐   (Enter number of times per day)
Forced Expiration ☐   y/n
Who does Physio ☐   1. Self   2. Parent   3. Both

	Dose Mg.	Frequency per day
Main oral antibiotic	☐	☐
Other oral antibiotic	☐	☐
Nebulized antibiotic	☐	☐
Bronchodilator & Method	☐	☐

Intal   y/n ☐
Beclomethasone   y/n ☐

Fat free Diet ☐   1. Strict   2. Relaxed   3. Free

Pancreatic Supplement ☐   1. Creon   2. Pancrease   3. Other

Dose per Meal ☐   Dose per Day ☐

Other Drugs ☐

CHO Supplement	☐ y/n	Vitamin E	☐ y/n
Protein Supplement	☐ y/n	MCT Oil	☐ y/n
Ketovite tabs	☐ y/n	Salt Tabs	☐ No. per Day
Ketovite liquid	☐ y/n	Calories/Kg/day	☐

EXAMINATION

Respiratory Rate per Minute ☐   Pulse ☐   Temp. ☐ C

Clubbing ☐   0. None   1. Nail bed hypertrophy   2. Watchglass   3. Drumstick

Chest Shape   0. Absent   1. Present   2. Severe

Sternal prominence ☐   Kyphosis ☐   Troughing ☐   Recession ☐

Auscultation

    Rhonchi ☐☐☐☐☐

    Crackles ☐☐☐☐☐

    Wheezing ☐☐☐☐☐

Breath Sounds ☐   0. Normal   1. Reduced

Pubertal Staging (1-5)

Breasts ☐   Pubic Hair ☐   Penis/Scrotum ☐   Testis vol. ☐ MI

Ears

Nose

Pharynx

Abdomen

Height Cm. ☐	FVC L. ☐	
Weight Kg. ☐	FVC% ☐	
FEV1 L. ☐	PEFR L. /s ☐	
FEV1% ☐	PEFR% ☐	

X-Ray done today? ☐   y/n

N-Crispin score Done? ☐   y/n

N-Crispin value ☐   (0-38)

Lung Score ☐

Anthropometric Score ☐

Date of last Sputum test ☐

Staph aureus present ☐   y/n

Pseudomonas present ☐   y/n

H. Influenzae present ☐   y/n

Other organism state

Sputum/Cough swab today ☐   y/n

Investigations:- Other

Changes in Management. . . . .

Summary. . . . .

. . . .

. . . .

. . . .

Seen by ☐   1. G. H.   2. M. S.   3. Registrar

Next visit in ☐   Weeks

The CF clinic: advantages and disadvantages

Advantages of a special CF clinic include improved health and life expectancy. A body of expert knowledge builds up and engenders confidence that the clinic is up to date with the latest advances in treatment. A camaraderie builds up between the children, their families and staff members, and there are improved research opportunities. Contact with subjects with more advanced disease and knowing affected people who die may be numbered among the disadvantages.

A question relating to CF clinics that is frequently asked is, 'Can one "catch" a *Pseudomonas* infection from someone else attending the clinic?' One very good study in Dublin has shown that only brothers and sisters tend to share the same *Pseudomonas* species. *Pseudomonas* is a very widespread micro-organism in nature, being found in any drainpipe, for instance. Person to person spread of the organism is likely to be of minor importance in CF.

Recent new methods of typing *Pseudomonas* strains, using differences in their genetic material shows that there is some cross-infection of *Pseudomonas aeruginosa* between patients, though this seems to be at a low level. In Copenhagen, Denmark, an attempt to keep people with *Pseudomonas* apart from those who were not yet colonized, resulted in a lower rate of infection. Recently at RMCH we have been alternating *Pseudomonas* and non-*Pseudomonas* clinic days. Cross-infection is much more likely to occur in confined spaces than in the open air and we have not changed our policy of taking children on camping holidays together, regardless of the *Pseudomonas* status.

A new phenomenon in some CF clinics is a related *Pseudomonas* species, *Pseudomonas cepacia*. This species does seem to have a slightly greater capacity to spread from person to person. In some Canadian clinics up to 40 per cent of patients are infected. The organism may occasionally be associated with a sudden deterioration in lung function and even death, but in many people the effect of *Pseudomonas cepacia* seems no different from that of *Pseudomonas aeruginosa*.

Specific aspects of CF management

Chest X-ray films are taken at least once a year. These are scored according to an accepted system to allow formal comparison. In addition, a Shwachman score is estimated yearly. This score gives points on the basis of well-being, school attendance, chest symptoms and signs, growth

Table 1. Clinical evaluation and grading criteria for patients with cystic fibrosis

Points	Case histories	Lungs, physical findings, and cough	Growth and nutrition	Chest X-ray
25	Full activity Normal exercise tolerance and endurance Normal strength Normal personality and disposition Normal school attendance	No cough Normal pulse and respiration No evidence of over-expansion Lungs clear to stethoscope Good posture No clubbing	Maintains weight and height well within normal range, or just like the rest of the family Good muscle development Normal amount of fat Normal sexual maturation Good appetite Well formed, almost normal stools	Normal
20	Slight limitation of strenuous activity Tires at end of day or after prolonged exertion Less energetic Low normal range of strength Occasionally irritable or lethargic Good school attendance	Occasional hacking cough Clearing of throat Resting pulse and respiration normal Mild over-expansion Occasional, usually localized, harsh breath sounds, wheezing or rattling mucus heard Good posture Mild clubbing	Maintains weight and height at slightly below average or the family normal Good muscle development Slightly decreased fat Slightly retarded sexual maturation Normal appetite Stools more frequent and slightly abnormal	Signs of excess air in slightly over-distended lungs

	General activity	Respiratory	Growth and nutrition	Chest X-ray
15	May rest voluntarily. Tires after exertion. Moderately inactive. Slight weakness. Lacking spontaneity. Lethargic or irritable. Fair school attendance	Mild chronic nonrepetitive cough in the morning on arising, after exertion or crying, or occasionally during the day. No night cough. Respiration and pulse *slightly* rapid. Barrel chest. Coarse breath sounds. Occasional localized mucus rattling or wheezing. Moderate rounding of shoulders. Moderate clubbing	Maintains weight and height at lower end of normal and less than other family members. Weight usually deficient for height. Fair muscle development. Moderately reduced fat. Abdomen slightly distended. Maturation definitely retarded. Fair appetite. Stools usually abnormal, large floating, occasionally foul, but formed	Excess air in over-distended lungs. Distance from front to back of chest increased. Diaphragm pushed down. Blood vessels in lungs prominent. Patches of lung with less air than normal
10	Limited physical activity and exercise tolerance. Breathless after exertion. Moderate weakness. Fussy, irritable, sluggish or listless. Poor school attendance, may require home tutor	Chronic cough, frequent, repetitive, productive and rarely paroxysmal. Respiration and pulse moderately rapid. Moderate to severe over-expansion. Widespread sounds of wheezing and mucus rattling	Weight and height below normal. Weight deficient for height. Poor muscle strength. Marked reduction in fat. Abdomen distended. Failure of sexual maturation and no adolescent growth spurt	As above, but more marked. Heart shadow narrow from pressure of lungs

Table 1. Clinical evaluation and grading criteria for patients with cystic fibrosis (*continued*)

Points	Case histories	Lungs, physical findings, and cough	Growth and nutrition	Chest X-ray
10 (ctd)		Rounded shoulders and forward head Marked clubbing Usually blueness of tongue	Poor appetite Stools poorly formed, bulky, fatty and foul smelling	
5	Severe limitations of activity Breathless when standing or lying down Inactive or confined to bed or chair Marked weakness Apathetic or irritable Cannot attend school	Severe paroxysmal, frequent productive cough, often associated with vomiting or blood in sputum Night cough Rapid pulse or respiration Marked barrel chest Generalized squeaking, bubbly noises and wheezing heard Poor posture Severe clubbing	Malnourished and stunted Weak, flabby, small muscles Absence of fat Large, flabby, protruberant abdomen Failure to grow or gain weight, often with weight loss Bulky, frequent, foul, fatty stools Frequent rectal prolapse	Marked overdistension Cystic spaces between areas of lung receiving too little air

This system of clinical evaluation can be used to evaluate patients at each visit or at six- or twelve-month intervals in order to determine the severity of the disease and the effect of therapy in any one patient and to compare one patient with the next.

The physical findings and chest X-ray are the best indicators of the degree of lung involvement and may be used without the other indicators to simplify and shorten the scoring. After Shwachman H. and Kukzycki L. T. (1958) Long term study of 105 patients with cystic fibrosis: studies made over a 5–14-year period. *Am J Dis Child*, **96**, 6–15.

and nutrition, and the X-ray results (see Table 1). Both scoring systems allow a more objective approach than is allowed by simply reacting to findings at any particular clinic visit. At RMCH we also perform occasional chest scans on patients. These involve injecting and inhaling safe radioactive substances into the body. These penetrate the air and blood supply of the patient's lungs. Photographic scans of the chest may then show areas of the lungs receiving too little air or blood (see Fig. 10). Such areas may not be detectable by X-rays or with a stethoscope. Lung changes cannot always be detected with the stethoscope, and this makes the occasional performance of these other tests necessary.

The different tests of lung function are fairly variable and are more useful as indicators of long-term changes rather than being immediately useful.

Lung function tests can, however, have immediate use in detecting a bronchospasm (contraction of the bronchial tubes). Sometimes bronchospasm may be suspected but cannot be detected with a stethoscope. In these circumstances, lung function tests are carried out before and after administration of a bronchodilator, a substance that relaxes the bronchial tubes. If bronchospasm is present, then the bronchodilator will improve the condition, and this will show on the second lung function tests. A bronchodilator drug can then be prescribed to ease the bronchospasm.

Inoculation

Inoculation against those organisms that cause respiratory illness is advisable in CF. In particular, this applies to measles and pertussis (whooping cough), and unless there are very strong reasons not to, these inoculations should be performed. Annual immunization against the prevalent influenza strain is worthwhile in those above the age of 4.

GENERAL ASPECTS OF CF TREATMENT

People with CF are encouraged to lead as normal and as active a life as possible. Children with CF who are swimming-fit, for instance, show improvement in their lung function and well-being. A cough is no bar to sporting activity, although, obviously, breathlessness does limit the activity of some. Experts in sports medicine are attached to some clinics.

Despite ignorance of the basic defect in CF, multi-disciplinary treatment has greatly prolonged life and its quality, so that reaching adulthood in reasonable health is becoming the rule rather than the exception.

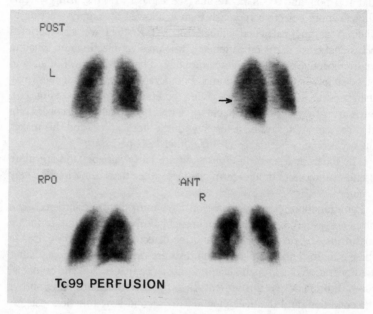

Fig. 10. A lung scan. Different panels show the lungs from different angles.

Perfusion tests are on the blood supply to various parts of the lung. Ventilation tests are on the distribution of inspired air to the various parts of the lung. Black areas on photographs are caused by radioactive emission. They denote lung tissue that is being well perfused or ventilated. White areas denote that the radioactive isotopes have not penetrated. Some of these areas are normal, and simply indicate the positions of the heart and spine. Other white areas denote parts of the lungs that are poorly perfused.

However, the severity of symptoms in individuals is highly variable, and very severely affected children may still die of the disease at a relatively young age, despite excellent treatment. More disturbing are patients who are initially only mildly affected but enter a more serious category simply through neglect of treatment.

Though there are many contributing factors, the improved survival in CF has been largely due to the development of effective antibiotics against *Staphylococcus* bacteria and to more effective treatment of *Pseudomonas* infections. Flucloxacillin and the more expensive fucidic acid are the most common antibiotics used to prevent and treat staphylococcal infections. There remain differences in practice between different clinics.

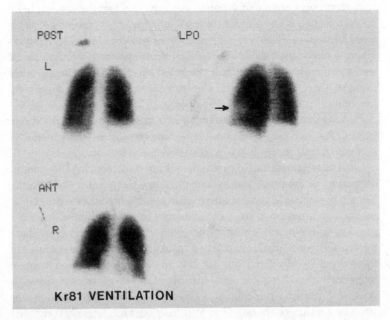

Fig. 10. (*cont.*) The two arrows in the figure mark an area of lung that is being poorly perfused and ventilated. This area was not obvious on listening to breathing with a stethoscope or on routine X-ray. Once found, special physiotherapy was applied to the particular zone.

Key: Tc99 = Technetium ⎫ radioactive isotopes that are inhaled (Tc99) or given by
     Kr81 = Krypton ⎭ injection (Kr81).

L	= left	POST	= posterior
R	= right	LPO	= left posterior oblique
ANT	= anterior	RPO	= right posterior oblique

Some, including ours at RMCH, believe in long-term (year-in, year-out) anti-staphylococcal treatment, using full therapeutic doses of either antibiotic mentioned above, given by mouth. We are able to eradicate the staphylococcal infection from the majority of our patients in this way. Other clinics prefer to treat a staphylococcal infection vigorously if it occurs. We believe that this can only be done safely in a CF clinic, with frequent testing for bacteria in sputum (phlegm) and careful surveillance. One danger of treating only the infection is that the family might not want to bother the doctor with a 'trivial' infection and some lung tissue damage may occur as a result of the delay in treatment.

A theoretical argument against long-term treatment of the staphylo-coccal infection is an idea that these bacteria may help prevent a *Pseudomonas* infection. There is no evidence to support this idea. Another question often raised about long-term treatment is whether the continual use of antibiotics can make these drugs less effective. Unlike many other bacteria, there is at present no evidence for *Staphylococcus* developing 'immunity' to the effects of antibiotics in CF.

Pseudomonas infections are difficult or impossible to eradicate. Once a mucoid *Pseudomonas* infection has become established it is generally a permanent feature, resulting in worsened lung function.

Current treatment can alleviate the infection by reducing the amount of sputum in the lungs and by keeping down the numbers of bacteria. Certain penicillins (e.g. azlocillin) together with aminoglycide drugs (e.g. netilmycin) are used to treat *Pseudomonas* infections. These drugs are given by injection into a vein. Other drugs that are sometimes used are the cephalosporins (e.g. ceftazidime), again given by injection. Courses of these drugs usually last about 10 days and are given in hospital where intensive physiotherapy and special attention to nutritional needs is possible. Sometimes these drugs or others (e.g. colomycin) that cannot be given by vein are given long-term by inhalation. One carefully controlled study of such inhalation in adults reported improved lung-function and well-being, with less days off work.

Difficulties of the treatment of pseudomonal infection are that most of the drugs used have to be given by injection, and the drugs may have unwelcome side-effects. However, it is rare to see the usual adverse effects on hearing and kidney function from these drugs in CF. Cipro-floxacin is an effective anti-*Pseudomonas* agent that can be taken by mouth and is thus rather attractive. However, bacteria become resistant to it fairly quickly (though they may sometimes regain their sensitivity). Treatment with ciprofloxacin may occasionally be complicated by severe joint pain in childhood. The pain disappears after a week or two of discontinuing the drug. Some way of rendering the conditions in the lung less ideal for the *Pseudomonas* bacteria would seem the only way of eradicating pseudomonal infections. One approach has been to vaccinate against the bacteria, but this has proved ineffective. Another experiment that was attempted involved removing free calcium from the mucus in the lungs (*Pseudomonas* bacteria are known to thrive when free calcium is available). Unfortunately, this approach was also unsuccessful.

Amiloride, a diuretic that blocks absorption of sodium ions, has been shown to partially correct the basic defect in the lung epithelium in CF.

As a result this drug was given by inhalation in an American trial. Though bronchial mucus was found to become thinner after its use and the agent was found to have a weak anti-bacterial effect, no dramatic improvement in the health of amiloride-treated CF patients occurred.

Cough suppressants or stimulants do not help CF patients with chest problems. This is because such compounds relieve symptoms but allow mucus to remain in the lungs, thus impairing their functions.

In some patients with CF, there is bronchospasm with wheezing. This may be associated with the CF or may be due to the very common chest condition, asthma. Bronchospasm in CF patients is treated in the same way as asthma. Inhalation of the drug cromoglycate may be used to prevent bronchospasm. On occasion bronchodilators (e.g. salbutamol) and steroids that act on the lung surface (e.g. beclamethasone) may be given to some patients by inhalation.

Very occasionally, the airways may be washed out under anaesthetic (bronchial lavage) in an attempt to clear accumulated secretions preventing aeration of parts of the lung. In extreme cases a segment of lung with permanently dilated bronchi may be surgically removed. In some CF clinics in the USA and Canada such treatments are undertaken rather more often than in Great Britain.

PHYSIOTHERAPY IN CF

A fit person breathes more efficiently than an unfit one, especially when exercising. Someone with CF who is fit and has 'trained' their respiratory muscles is able to cope with the stresses of a chest infection more easily than an unfit person. The need for this 'training' may be especially marked in girls, since their muscles are often less well developed than those of boys. This is partly because of true sex differences in muscle bulk and strength, but differences are also partly cultural, with girls tending to play less active games inside, while boys are often more active outside. Girls with CF do slightly less well than boys at any age, and this may be partly because of weak chest muscles. This situation can be remedied by an active approach to physical exercise which develops the chest, especially swimming. People with CF who become swimming fit show an improvement in lung function.

It is precisely when the child is well that physiotherapy and chest muscle training are important. Some children and parents seem to think that paying attention to physiotherapy when the child has a cough is sufficient. Mucus in CF is relatively dehydrated, but if there is infection and the bronchi are dilated, secretions of mucus and sputum can be very copious. Clearance of these secretions is paramount in allowing maximal ventilation of the lungs. Young children swallow their sputum, so the fact that none is being coughed out does not mean that no sputum is being produced.

In CF the upper lobes of the lungs are particularly prone to attack, although the reasons for this are unknown. The techniques employed in improving the strength and efficiency of the muscles of respiration and the clearing of sputum include breathing exercises (see p. 50), chest clapping with cupped hands, sitting or lying in various positions to help mucus drainage (see Fig. 11). The paediatrician may direct the attention of the physiotherapist and the parents to an area that requires special attention, because of physical signs found on examining the chest, or on an X-ray or scan. All CF patients are taught the forced expiration technique (FET), whereby the person breathes out in short, powerful huffs. The method has been shown to result in improved lung functions, and has the great advantage of allowing older people a greater degree of freedom, since it reduces the need for another person to help with the physiotherapy.

Inhalation of bronchodilators may be prescribed for use at or near the beginning of a physiotherapy session. Inhaled antibiotics are also taken as part of the physiotherapy session, but *at the end* (otherwise, of course, much of the antibiotic would be coughed up in the sputum and lost).

The hospital-based physiotherapist, the parents, and the child are the

---

Fig. 11. Positions for postural (bronchial) drainage. This series of illustrations shows the best positions for drainage of mucus from various parts of the lung. (All illustrations redrawn from Library of Congress Publication No. 74-21835, Cystic Fibrosis Foundation.)

(a) Diagram showing the various lobes of the lung.
(b) Postures for drainage of upper lobes of lung. (i) Apical segments; (ii) anterior segments; (iii) posterior segments.
(c) Drainage postures for lower lobes of lung. (i) Superior segments; (ii) anterior basal segments; (iii) lateral basal segments; (iv) posterior basal segments.
(d) Posture for drainage of lingular segments of left upper lobe.
(e) Drainage posture for right middle lobe of lung.
(f) Two positions in which the individual can perform self-therapy. (i) Upper lobe of lung, posterior segment. (ii) Right middle lobe of lung.

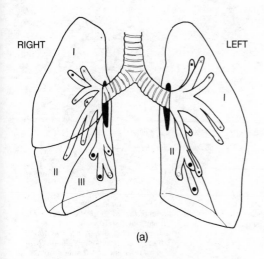

Key:
- ▪ I Upper lobe
- × 1. Apical
- ＊ 2. Anterior
- ■ 3. Posterior
- ＋ II 4–R Middle lobe – 4–L Lingula
  III Lower lobe
- ▲ 5. Superior
- • 6. Anterior basal
- ● 7. Lateral basal
-    8. Posterior basal

RIGHT   LEFT

(a)

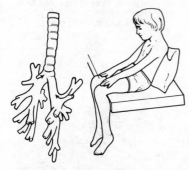

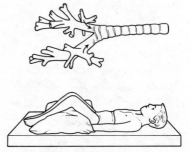

(i) Bed or drainage table flat. Patient leans back on pillow at 30° angle against therapist. Therapist claps with markedly cupped hand over area between clavicle (collarbone) and top of scapula (shoulder blade) on each side.)

(ii) Bed or drainage table flat . Patient lies back with pillow under knees. Therapist claps between clavicle (collarbone) and nipple on each side.

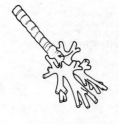

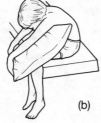

(iii) Bed or drainage table flat. Patient leans over folded pillow at 30° angle. Therapist stands behind and claps over upper back on both sides.

(b)

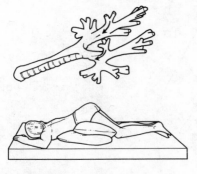

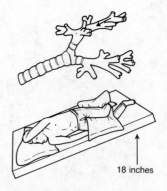

(i) Bed or table flat. Patient lies on abdomen with two pillows under hips. Therapist claps over middle of back at tip of scapula (shoulder blade), on either side of spine.

(ii) Foot of table or bed elevated 18 inches (about 30°). Patient lies on side, head down, pillow under knees. Therapist claps with slightly cupped hand over lower ribs. (Position shown is for drainage of *left* anterior basal segment. To drain the right anterior basal segment, patient should lie on his left side in same posture.)

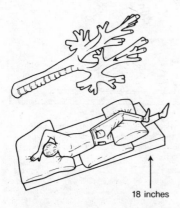

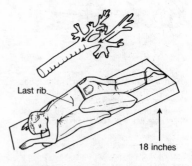

(iii) Foot of table or bed elevated 18 inches (about 30°). Patient lies on abdomen, head down, then rotates ¼ turn upward. Upper leg is flexed over pillow for support. Therapist claps over uppermost portion of lower ribs. (Position shown is for drainage of *right* lateral basal segment. To drain the left lateral basal segment, patient should lie on his right side in the same posture.)

(iv) Foot of table or bed elevated 18 inches (about 30°). Patient lies on abdomen, head down, with pillow under hip. Therapist claps over lower ribs close to spine on each side.

(c)

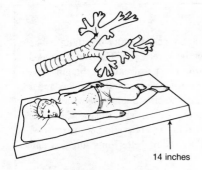

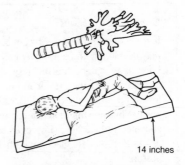

Foot of table or bed elevated 14 inches (about 15°). Patient lies head down on right side and rotates ¼ turn backward. Pillow may be placed behind from shoulder to hip. Knees should be flexed. Therapist claps with moderately cupped hand over left nipple area. In females with breast developed or tenderness, use cupped hand with heel of hand under armpit and fingers extending forward beneath the breast.

(d)

Foot of table or bed elevated 14 inches (about 15°). Patient lies head down on left side and rotates ¼ turn backward. Pillow may be placed behind from shoulder to hip. Knees should be flexed. Therapist claps over right nipple area. In females with breast development or tenderness, use cupped hand with heel of hand under armpit and fingers extending forward beneath the breast.

(e)

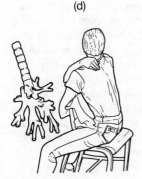

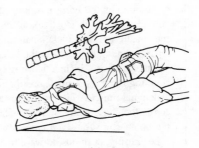

(i) Lean forward over back of chair on folded pillow at about 30° angle. Clap with cupped hand and vibrate over upper back extending fingers forward and upward.

(f)

(ii) Foot of bed elevated 10–14 inches about 15° angle. Lie on left side ¼ turn, head down (pillow behind from shoulder to hip), knees flexed. Clap and vibrate over right nipple.

team that look after physiotherapy needs. In some CF clinics the physiotherapist forms the closest relationship of all with the parents. What does require discipline on the part of all, is to realize the often progressive nature of the condition, which may deteriorate despite meticulous attention to all aspects of treatment.

Breathing exercises

If the upper and lower airways become blocked, faulty breathing habits may develop, with poor movement of the lower chest. The over-expanded lungs may reduce the mobility of the chest wall and diaphragm. The increased effort may result in poor posture, with round shoulders and a forward position of the head. Breathing exercises improve ventilation and posture by allowing more efficient use of the diaphragm and muscles of the abdomen in breathing. Improved breathing and relaxation of the muscles of the upper chest, neck, and shoulders allow better lung function and posture.

A summary of a good breathing exercise follows.

Place one hand on the upper chest and one on the abdomen. Breathe in deeply through the nose—the abdomen should rise but the upper chest should remain still. Breathe out slowly with the lips pursed, making the sound 'pff'—this increases the pressure inside the airways and prevents them from collapsing too soon in expiration. Note that the abdomen has become flat. The out breath should take three times as long as the in breath.

The exercise described above can be done lying flat or sitting in a chair with the back well supported. If done sitting, one bends over during expiration. In the lying position, placing of a book or graded weights (anything from 1 lb to 10 lb) on the abdomen provides an extra load for the diaphragm and abdominal muscles to move and increases their strength and bulk, much as the biceps are developed using a barbell.

Other exercises include blowing bubbles, balloons, candle flames, and counting games on a single breath. Sit-ups are excellent for strengthening abdominal muscles. Lie on your back on the floor; with the arms folded across the chest, come slowly to a sitting position. Try to daily increase the number of sit-ups you are able to do before tiring.

Leg raising, push-ups, forward bends, and weight-lifting strengthen the shoulder and abdominal muscles.

The stronger all these muscles are, the easier coughing becomes. Abdominal pain from frequent or deep coughing is thus lessened. Breathing exercises are specially important in girls, who tend to have less well developed musculature.

NUTRITIONAL AND DIETARY ASPECTS

There are increased energy requirements in CF. This is particularly so in those with advanced lung disease where sometimes food intake cannot match the body's needs and there is progressive weight loss. With older pancreatic enzyme preparations, steatorrhoea (fatty diarrhoea) was a problem, and many children took less than the optimal amount of food to reduce the amount of strong flatus and foul-smelling stools. When the new pancreatic enzyme preparations, Pancrease® and Creon®, were introduced, food absorption became much more efficient and stools returned to normal appearance. Many people with CF remained on their restricted diet at first. It was only when the concept of a normal diet, providing about 130 per cent (i.e. substantially more than the usual intake) of protein, fat, and carbohydrate, but with sufficient enzyme capsules to allow normal absorption, was introduced that normal nutrition became available for all those without advanced lung disease. The amount of new pancreatic enzyme capsules, sometimes as many as 20 with a meal has become an inconvenience, much as was high dosage with the older pancreatic enzyme preparations. Drug firms are hoping to introduce more concentrated capsules with higher lipase to further reduce the number needed. It is thought that good nutrition protects to an extent against the progress of lung disease. The hope is that such dietary treatment given from childhood will result in an overall significant increase in health in adulthood and, in turn, increased longevity.

Some people with CF find it difficult to take sufficient calories for their nutritional requirements in a normal high energy diet. Night feeding of high calorie and energy protein–fat hydrolysates given during sleep by drip, using a fine polythene tube passed via the nose, gullet, and thence into the stomach have helped many to gain weight. Many of those people with CF who have used this way of feeding are very pleased with it and there are children of primary-school age who have learned to pass their own tubes. The treatment is not recommended for those with recurrent night coughing, since in these circumstances the tube could become coughed out of position with the danger of food entering the lungs.

Even more efficient night feeding may be achieved by gastrostomy, a minor operation in which a soft, fairly large-bore tube is inserted into the stomach through the left side of the abdomen. This route may be used over a period of many months or even years, although the tube needs to be replaced from time to time. The newer technique of 'button' gastrostomy has fewer side effects. The views of one of our patients, Michael who is 14 and of his parents will give some insights into what such an operation means to a patient and his family.

Michael's view of gastrostomy:

As a CF sufferer one of my problems was poor weight-gain. Although the dietician and doctors had tried for many years to get me to put on weight, nothing seemed to work especially as my appetite was very, very poor. I didn't have much energy and as a result I didn't feel like joining in anything. Also, my chest was quite bad.

The day of my operation I was rather scared, even though everyone concerned had explained as much as they could about what was going to happen to me. When I awoke from the anaesthetic after the operation, I felt groggy and very sore around my stomach. To make matters worse, a bit later that day I had to have physiotherapy, which wasn't very pleasant. In order to keep my chest clear I have to have physio quite often. Gradually I recovered from the operation, and was walking around in a couple of days. At this stage I felt maybe I shouldn't have had the gastrostomy.

The first tube that was inserted through my stomach and came out through my abdomen was very thick, long, and rigid. It was extremely sore and uncomfortable. Before the tube was put in I was told that it would be quite flexible and I would be able to do most things I had managed to do before. This was not entirely true and I had problems. I asked the surgeon if it would be possible to have a softer, more flexible tube put in. This was agreed and happily I did not need another operation for this to be done (I was simply given a relaxant while the surgeon changed the tube). Although I have now had 9 tubes inserted in turn, looking back it was all worthwhile, as I have gained 2 stones in weight and have also grown taller. I feel much better and I would highly recommend a gastrostomy to any fellow CF sufferer who had difficulty gaining weight.

Next, the view of Michael's parents:

At the time it was suggested that Michael might benefit from the gastrostomy operation, his appetite and weight were very poor. This had been a problem for a number of years and although the doctors, dietician, and everyone concerned had tried hard it was to no avail. He was 14 years old and weighed just 5 stone.

After visiting the clinic and being told what the operation entailed, we went home to discuss it with Michael. This was not easy, particularly since Michael would be the first CF patient at the RMCH to be considered for this operation. As a result we had no other CF parent or patient to look to in this matter. If we did decide to agree to the operation all we could do was to put our trust in the medical team. After a few days, we decided that Michael should have the gastrostomy, but we were all very apprehensive.

After his operation Michael was understandably very sore, and post-operative physiotherapy was a problem because every time he had to cough up sputum it was very painful. However, he made a fairly quick recovery, though there were times when we wondered if we had done the right thing.

It is now nearly a year since the gastrostomy was performed and he looks and feels so much better. Michael now weighs 7 stone and to date is doing well, although it has not been all plain sailing. He has needed to have quite a number of new tubes inserted, as they do tend to wear thin. This doesn't entail any more operations but it does mean having the inconvenience of having to get to the hospital as soon as possible.

Along with everything else that needs to be done for a CF child (or in our case a CF teenager): for example, physiotherapy and administering medication, we now have to mix a feed for the gastrostomy tube. At night, the feed is gradually given to Michael by the tube with the aid of a Kangaroo pump. The dressings around the tube have to be changed daily, but this has really become part of our general routine. If anyone wants to know if we feel it was all worthwhile, as a family living and coping with it, the answer is 'Yes'! The benefit of seeing Michael in so much better health really does make it all worthwhile.

Where undernutrition is a serious problem there may be a limited success with nutrients given by vein. During treatment there may be weight-gain and an improvement in the chest disease. The treatment can sometimes have a role in those being prepared for heart–lung transplants. Many physicians make use of the periods required in hospital for the intravenous treatment of chest infections to give some extra nutrition by vein. In a recent experimental trial, 12 volunteers were given a diet consisting of soya oil, amino acids, and glucose at 130 per cent of normal daily intake level for 2–3 weeks. The diet was given entirely by vein. Those given the treatment showed weight-gain that was still retained 6 months later, significantly fewer chest infections, and improved lung function. By its nature, this study could not be performed in a scientifically controlled way; that is, it was not possible to give another group of patients other substances intravenously for comparison.

Occasional patients persist with steatorrhoea despite huge doses of pancreatic enzymes. In some of these patients an elegant group of drugs that reduce the amount of acid produced by the stomach and aid its emptying, may result in improved absorption of food in the gut. (Examples of these drugs are cimetidine and ranitidine.) Although such drugs are effective in treating people with peptic ulcers, it does not seem desirable in CF to interfere with the normal working of the stomach over long periods of time, so their use is limited to special situations.

Pancreatic enzymes

Preparations of pancreatic enzymes from pigs have been used for many years to supplement the digestive enzymes of CF patients. Older preparations were largely inactivated in the stomach by acid, when the gelatin of the capsule containing the enzymes was digested away. Specially covered enteric-coated tablets, which are not broken down by stomach acids, passed through the duodenum before the whole of the enteric coating was lost. Hence the enzymes contained in the tablets had passed the site at which they were needed (the duodenum) before they were released. It was only when enteric-coated microspheres or microgranules were introduced that adequate amounts of the enzymes were released in the alkaline milieu of the duodenum. It is at this site that normal pancreatic enzymes released by the body would meet the bolus of food from the stomach.

In infants and young children, too young to swallow capsules, care should be given to give microgranules from opened capsules with acidic rather than alkaline foods. We have found that giving granules with apple sauce at the start, in the middle, and at the end of the feed or meal works best. Because of its alkaline pH, milk is not an ideal vehicle.

Today, virtually all people with CF take one of the newer enteric-coated microgranule pancreatic preparations: Pancrease® or Creon®. Larger and larger amounts of enzyme have been prescribed to allow a completely unrestricted diet. The number of capsules taken with meals once again threatens to become inconvenient, but undoubtedly nutrition, at least until puberty, in CF has been greatly improved by the approach of a large number of enzyme capsules and an unrestricted diet aimed at providing 130 per cent of normal nutritional needs.

Salt

There are increased salt needs in CF, particularly in hot weather. Certain children seem particularly prone to acute salt depletion and the need for extra salt should be considered in any child with CF who shows signs of lethargy. Occasionally, during a heatwave, a child may become weak or dehydrated and may need saline solution to be given intravenously. Dietary salt is often cited as a cause of high blood pressure, but in CF this is not the case, because increased salt in the sweat provides a safety mechanism.

Vitamins

Because of the malabsorption of fat in CF, the fat-soluble vitamins A, D, E, and K are taken by most people with the disease. There does not seem a good reason to challenge this practice, although the necessity of yet more tablets is inconvenient. There is evidence from blood tests that people with CF suffer from vitamin D deficiency, but the disease that results when there is such a deficiency, rickets, has never been described in CF. A group of CF adults in Birmingham who also suffered from ataxia (a disorder of balance) were shown to be vitamin E deficient, and the ataxia symptoms disappeared when vitamin E was administered. Night blindness from vitamin A deficiency has been described in CF.

Trace elements

Some elements, such as iron, selenium, and zinc are found in very small amounts in the body. They are necessary for certain body functions (for example, iron is an integral part of haemoglobin, the molecule that transports oxygen around the blood), and must therefore be taken in the diet. No deficiencies of zinc, selenium, or iron have been found in people with CF.

TREATMENT OF OTHER SYMPTOMS OF CF

Meconium ileus equivalent

An increased dosage of pancreatic enzymes is the first approach to treating this condition. Surgical treatment of meconium ileus equivalent may occasionally be necessary, but most attacks can be managed by increasing liquid intake and by administering water-attracting enemas (e.g. Gastrographin®) or drugs like acetyl cysteine (which thins the intestinal mucus). (Attempts to use the mucus-thinning properties of acetyl cysteine to treat lung complications in CF have proved fruitless, as the action of the drug was found to be too vigorous).

Rectal prolapse in infancy comes under control once the steatorrhoea is treated.

Diabetes

As mentioned earlier, the diabetes in CF is generally mild and small doses of insulin suffice to control it. There are generally some modifications needed in the diet, and a diabetic with CF would need to ensure that salt intake was adequate. We at RMCH generally share the care of diabetic CF patients with a diabetes specialist.

Varices

It was explained in Chapter 2 (p. 25) how varices or dilated veins occur at the lower end of the gullet in people with cirrhosis of the liver. People with varices must avoid taking aspirin or similar substances, as these drugs may cause bleeding. Individuals with varices may need to take vitamin K and drugs of the cimetidine group to reduce stomach acid. Occasionally, sclerosing agents may be needed. These drugs strengthen the walls of the blood vessels, thus making bleeding less likely. These are injected directly into the varices, under anaesthetic.

FERTILITY AND CF

Adults with CF often ask for counselling about fertility. Nearly all men with CF are sterile and their ejaculate contains no sperm. Nevertheless, in a small percentage of cases this is not so, and men with CF have been known to father children. Women with CF are fertile, though they may have abnormal cervical mucus and may sometimes come to infertility clinics. Some women are not well enough to be able to undertake pregnancies, but an increasing number of women with CF are having children.

Pregnancy

Sadly, the cost of pregnancy is great for women with CF. Heart failure may occur, and lung function often deteriorates. In the only good study of its kind, 18 of 100 women who undertook pregnancies were dead within two years of giving birth, with 12 of them dying within six months. The chances of the baby dying within a few days of birth and of being premature were also increased in this group. Other factors that deserve consideration are the impact of the mother's shorter lifespan on the offspring and the possible inability of the mother to see to the child's daily needs. It is generally agreed that unless the disease is very mild, women with CF are best advised to avoid pregnancy.

Contraception

Oral contraceptives should be used with great care by women with CF, as they can cause blood clots in the veins. Oral contraceptives should be particuarly avoided when there is liver damage (as in cirrhosis). For many women with CF, spermicidal jelly in conjunction with condoms is the method of choice.

The foregoing are many of the general aspects that might be dealt with when genetic counselling in CF is given. Specific details of tests of prenatal diagnosis are discussed in chapter 6.

4

Heart–lung transplants and cystic fibrosis

A great deal of publicity has been given to the combined heart–lung transplant as a means of increasing the lifespan of children and the growing number of young adults with CF. Obviously this operation is only going to be available to a relatively small percentage of CF patients. There are still only a small number of centres in the UK with the expertise and facilities to carry out this major feat of surgery. Since these centres are also carrying out operations on all other relevant medical cases, the CF patients must take their turn on a long waiting list. Even when an individual has entered the transplant programme, having fulfilled all the necessary criteria, it may be a very long wait before he or she can be transplanted. The major delay, of course, is the shortage of donor organs. When a donor is identified it is then really down to the luck of the draw as to who on the waiting list has the same blood group (hence reducing the chances of rejection of the transplanted organs) and organs of about the same size of the donor.

If two potential recipients are equally well matched to a donor, then a clinical decision as to which of the two is sicker and hence more in need of the transplant, will be made.

It must also be said that not all heart–lung transplant patients survive the operation nor the immediate problems of infection and organ rejection. Furthermore, we still do not know by how long this operation is capable of prolonging the life of a CF patient. Since the operation is a relatively new one, only time will answer the question. In other words, in the absence of effective treatment for the terminally ill CF patients who have entered the stage of lung failure, it is reasonable to attempt this relatively high-risk operation. However, it is hoped that in the longer term, as the major advances in our understanding of CF that will follow on from the isolation of the CF gene (see p. 10) are transmitted into an effective treatment for lung disease, this operation may be superseded.

Clive Sandercock and Gary Gifford are two of the CF patients who have received combined heart–lung transplants and more than 9 months after their operations they spoke to one of the authors (A.H.) about it.

Gary is now 23; he was diagnosed as having CF at the age of 18 months. As a child he was often sick, being in and out of hospital frequently until the age of 12 or 13. From then until he was around 18 things went rather better, but the next two years saw a relatively rapid deterioration in his health, and by the time he was 21 he was more or less unable to do anything that expended energy. He had actually been an in-patient at the Brompton Hospital in London for more than 3 months, relying on a continual oxygen supply to survive before he received his transplant.

Clive is 30, has a relatively mild form of CF with no digestive system involvement. An infection caught on holiday at the age of 14 turned into a severe chest infection which led to the diagnosis of CF being made. Even though from this age onwards he always had a cough and was frequently short of breath, it never seriously impeded his life and his job as a mechanic. However, from the age of 25 or 26 his health deteriorated quite rapidly. He was in the Brompton Hospital for 7 weeks before having the transplant. Clive has a much rarer blood group than Gary and fortuitously a matched donor became available relatively soon. Though more potential donors with Gary's blood group became available, there were obviously more patients with the same type on the waiting list above him.

Both Clive and Gary described the wait for the operation, once they knew they had been placed on the list, as by far the worst part of the whole procedure.

Before the operation you know that every day you are going to get a little bit worse and after it you are going to get a little bit better. Even very soon after the operation you could start doing things that you wouldn't have thought of doing beforehand, little things that to most people would seem like nothing but to yourself are big steps forward. For example, brushing your teeth. Before the transplant you just didn't have enough puff to do this, you would do three brush-strokes and then stop because you had run out of energy. Now, you just brush your teeth without thinking about it.

Another difficult time was actually coming up to the Brompton Hospital, otherwise known as the National Heart and Lung Hospital, in the centre of London. Clive said that this was really quite a shock and he felt rather lost, too far away from home surroundings (both Clive and Gary come from the Cornwall and Devon areas), and that until he came to accept this move it was pretty tough going. To add to the problems at this stage, Clive was feeling really ill and his condition deteriorated over the next few weeks in the Brompton. He had so little energy that he was unable even to walk around his bed. Not only did lack of oxygen make him look blue but it also made him behave in slightly crazy ways, doing things which he later regretted, but which he was often not aware of doing at the time. For example, pulling out his catheters, and being aggressive to the nursing staff and doctors. Behaviour like this is certainly not in his nature!

Until the last few weeks before his operation Gary had tried to go outside for a short walk each day. He set himself something to look forward to every day and a challenge to meet, however small, even if it was only to walk up the hospital corridor. During his last few weeks at the Brompton he could not leave his hospital room, and he knew he never would without a transplant (he was on a continual oxygen supply and had no energy to move). He recalls that some days he felt so terribly ill that he could have given up and died, but that he made himself fight on.

The heart–lung transplant operations were performed at Harefield Hospital in Middlesex. Both Clive and Gary described the move to Harefield Hospital as 'great'. They were both warned that although a suitable organ donor had become available, it was at that stage far from certain that the operation would go ahead. Despite this, the overwhelming feeling was one of relief that at last the wait was over and that now they were going to have a chance of a successful operation. As Clive said: 'As long as I got to Harefield's and they did something then at least I had had my chance and it was my own fight after that.'

The actual heart–lung transplant operation obviously does not feature prominently in their memory of the whole story. Both had seen a video describing what was going to happen to them. When they actually first registered all that was going on around them (remarkably soon) after the surgery, they were surprised by how few external signs there were of what had just happened to them. The intricate machinery of monitors, catheters, blood bottles, and so on that are part of such a major operation were all hidden, either behind the bed-head or under the bed. All they could see were a few pacer wires attached to their body, and they did not even have a long line of stitches in their chest, the incision having been closed by laser 'stitching'. Of course, although their parents had been warned what they would see from the other end of the bed, they were still pretty shocked.

Clive remarked that though it was uncomfortable and they both felt rather 'beaten up and sore' after the surgery, they never actually felt any major pain associated with it. In fact, their arms and shoulders were very sore from the actual physical trauma they had suffered during the long operation. Their major worry at this stage was not disturbing their new set of organs by moving too violently or breaking open their wound during physiotherapy. It took Clive and Gary quite a long time to get fit again after the heart–lung transplant, mainly because they had been so ill for a long period before the operation. Their muscles were already wasted, they were very thin, and even lying in bed made them sore. Both spent 5 weeks in Harefield Hospital after the operation, and then several weeks in a flat in Harefield village which allowed them to be fully independent but yet to have the safety net of the hospital nearby, particularly during the early stages when rejection of the new organs can first become a major problem.

Gary describes his life after the heart–lung transplant as 'brilliant'! 'I've never had it so good, I'm doing all sorts of things that I haven't been able to do for years and never thought I would be able to do again.' He plays table tennis and five-a-side football. They are both *so* happy to be able to lead a relatively normal life again: to be able to get up in the morning, get dressed and start their day rather than spending hours 'getting ready', doing physiotherapy, and so on; to be able to run down the road to get the morning paper rather than planning their trip to the paper shop round where and how often they could stop for a rest; to have the ability to take the stairs rather than having to use the adjacent escalator. They feel that their social lives are better because they have so much more self confidence.

Clive and Gary both admit that things have not been completely straightforward since their operation and that maybe they sometimes paint too rosy a picture. They do still get days when they don't feel well, but even when this happened soon after the transplant they could see that every day they were able to achieve something they could not do before. For the first few weeks they had a great deal of nausea and Gary suffered from fluid build-up, which put pressure on his lungs and liver. They were very apprehensive about the symptoms and side-effects of the operation, worrying that they might be signs of organ rejection. They suffered some depression, particularly when they felt they were not recovering as fast as some other heart–lung transplant patients had. An early worry also was whether or not the new pair of lungs was going to start deteriorating in function, as their own pair had done. They were encouraged to cough and clear their lungs, just as if they were doing characteristic physiotherapy for CF treatment. However, it now seems that, at least so far, their transplanted lungs are not showing any CF-related disease.

Several months later, they see the only major side-effects of their treatment as the continual need for immunosuppressant drugs (to prevent organ rejection) and the effects of steroids. The most noticeable feature of steroid intake is the marked effect it has in promoting the growth of hair, both on the face and the body. Obviously, though the young men do not mind this, it can be quite upsetting for young women.

When asked to summarize the most important attributes for a CF patient who is going to enter the heart–lung transplant programme, Clive and Gary homed in on the same points. First, they need a really positive attitude to life, and second, they need a solid family back-up. As Clive said, 'When you feel rough you have to think: I've got to keep going, I've got to hang in there and wait; you must never think "I'd rather be dead". You need a lot of parental support and support from your friends to keep going.' In fact, both were sure they would not have got through the whole thing without parental support, and that it was actually more difficult for their parents than it was for them. Their parents felt so helpless, watching their son going downhill fast, and then unable to contribute during the operation and recovery period, while at least Clive and Gary could contribute in a 'mind over matter' sense. Neither feels that opting for the chance of an operation that is so obviously risky and traumatic as a heart–lung transplant was a courageous decision. They felt so ill before the operation and knew that they were going to die, so that given any chance to feel better and prolong their life, they had to take it. As Gary said, 'I've always enjoyed life, even when I was feeling bad, and I so much wanted to live I just had to go for the operation.'

5

Psychology of cystic fibrosis

Many aspects of the disease CF, its chronic nature, uncertainties about long-term prognosis, the genetic aspects, and the impact on family life, to name but a few, can affect the psychological functioning of the affected person, individual family members, and the family as a whole.

The experienced CF clinic team can play an important role in recognizing early signs of psychological difficulties and in providing support and advice. Sometimes difficulties may be so marked that the Paediatrician may call on the expertise of the team's Clinical Psychologist.

People with CF, and their families, tend to be realistic about their situation and to cope with day-to-day and long-term problems. It does need to be emphasized that the illness itself and its treatment does impose a life-long discipline on the individual and the family.

Cystic fibrosis affects people with widely differing temperaments and from diverse backgrounds. The reactions of various family members tend to depend more on these factors than on the CF condition itself. This said, there are specific occasions in the evolution of the CF when stress factors may be increased:

At the time of diagnosis

Since most diagnoses are made in early infancy or childhood, it is the parents who first experience psychological distress. The anxiety and frustration at the months of frequent visits to the doctor with complaints about their child's abnormal stools or recurrent cough may surface when the diagnosis is finally made. The relief that a diagnosis has finally been made is often tempered by the stark realization of what the diagnosis may imply. In earlier times, couples tended never to have heard of CF until the doctor presented them with the diagnosis in their child. Mass media (magazines, TV, radio) attention to CF will often mean that individuals have heard of the disorder, and often about some dramatic (newsworthy) aspect. Thus alarm at the diagnosis may be their first reaction.

Occasionally the diagnosis may have been missed for years. Then frustration and anger may be especially keenly felt, aggravated by fear of a worsened prognosis because of the delay.

Rejection of the accuracy of the diagnosis by the parents is seldom a problem where diagnostic tests were performed after the child became ill. However, diagnoses which follow on screening tests and with the child still healthy can understandably be challenged by parents, though the onset of symptoms is seldom long delayed.

The CF team is careful not to overwhelm parents with too much knowledge about the condition too quickly, and is available to provide a great deal of support in the early days. Frequent clinic and home visits enable parents to develop confidence about CF, its treatment and the long-term outlook.

Meconium ileus

Here there has been no delay in making the diagnosis. However, a dramatic operation within a few days of the child's birth, with the baby sometimes in an Intensive Care Unit far away from home, causes its own stresses.

We know of couples who have been left with the abiding feeling that they could cope with a second child affected by CF but not with a second operation in the newborn period for meconium ileus. The nurse from the CF team is increasingly called by the intensive care surgical team to make the first contacts with the parents, to instil confidence about the future.

Childhood

Most young children with CF need to spend very little time in hospital, and require a minimum of injections. With better nutrition and improved pancreatic enzymes most will not stand out from their peers. However, for those who are more severely affected there may be problems with being underweight, with the recurrent severe cough and with time off school. For some, with early *Pseudomonas* infection, there is the pain and discomfort of hospital admission and of the intravenous needles needed for antibiotic administration. Some children may be embarrassed by the number of pancreatic enzyme capsules they need to take with their school meals. Children have been known to discard or conceal their capsules. Some young children may rebel against their enforced inactivity during physiotherapy sessions, and elicit anxiety in their mother or father. Visits to the CF clinic may be times of stress for the parents, worried that some sign of deterioration may be found or that their fears in this regard may be confirmed. On the other hand, there is usually the reassurance that the check-up, discussion of problems, and adjustments in treatment brings, so parents and child often go home relieved that the situation is under control. Failure to keep appointments at the CF clinic is always treated seriously by the team, and may sometimes signify a psychological problem. Friendships between families develop at clinic or through CF organizations. News travels fast between some of the families about dramatic events, such as someone dying of CF or a heart–lung transplant that has occurred. Such events can explain temporarily increased levels of anxiety.

Adolescence

Adolescents with CF are no different from other adolescents in terms of concerns about the future, their looks, relationships with the opposite sex, etc. It is also a period of emerging independence, when peer groups can be important. Parents rightly worry when an adolescent becomes rebellious and rejecting of treatment. Some adolescents may ask pertinent questions about their disease and begin to be more forceful in their views about treatment. This may involve requests for more home versus hospital intravenous antibiotic courses. They may express concerns about long-term survival, and the boys about sterility. Some adolescents may lag far behind their peers in terms of height and weight—this is especially, though not only, in the presence of advanced lung disease. People in this group may be prepared to undergo the inconvenience of nightly naso-gastric or gastrostomy feeding to increase the amount of calories taken in. Being underweight and undersized may dominate their thoughts (see Michael's comments in Chapter 3).

Adulthood

There is a great camaraderie among many adults through the Associations for CF Adults. These articulate groups have vocalized some of the concerns and needs of affected adults and have helped many professionals understand their problems. Having a job is as important to the dignity and self-esteem of a person with CF as it is to any other person in our society. One dilemma which adults may face is whether to mention their disease to employers. According to the Association for Cystic Fibrosis

Adults, 50 per cent of affected adults in Britain are employed, 18 per cent unemployed, and 3.6 per cent unable to work through illness. Of the remainder, about half are students and half housewives.

Reactions of individual adults to their illness differ widely. Some few regard the CF as a treasured part of their personality, while most regard the CF as a challenge, trying not to let the disease dominate their lives.

Relatively few men with CF marry (10 per cent), while 33 per cent of women do. Both sexes do form long-standing relationships. Perhaps the implications of being sterile may be a reason for the low marriage rate in males.

Affected women who decide not to have children need to consider sterilization as a preferred mode of contraception. Couples who decide that they do want children have to consider this option very carefully for a number of reasons, including the possible effects on the woman's health. An affected man and his wife may wish to have a child, using donor sperm. It would be important to ensure that the donor is not a CF carrier.

The Adult Association accepts the issue of prenatal diagnosis and termination of a pregnancy with CF as a matter of personal conscience. Understandably, this is a sensitive area.

The impact of new treatments

Most dramatic of these has been heart–lung transplant. The great majority of parents and of affected children or adults are positive about wishing to accept the offer when it is made. A prelude to this is the conversation with the doctor about the hopeless long-term prognosis without surgery. This conversation, however difficult, used to be the one to help the parents and child to prepare for the child's death. Now the offer of curative treatment may dominate this phase, and there needs to be counselling, generally undertaken by the transplant team, about the fine details of the procedure and preparation for it. For some there is the happy outcome of a successful transplant, for others death comes with the person still on a waiting list and sometimes with inadequate preparation. The CF team needs to exercise its medical and psychological skills to the full in helping the affected person and the family to cope with any outcome.

There is the comfort that everything possible was tried, which may help the parents to get over their grief, if the person does die. Not all those who have transplants survive, and it is difficult for the parents and

CF team to remember that an 80 per cent survival chance includes a 20 per cent chance of failure. One additional source of pride to individuals and families may be the so-called domino procedure, where the heart of the CF sufferer is used in heart transplant while he or she receives a heart–lung transplant from another donor. The various difficulties still attendant on transplant are seen as an inevitable price for true progress.

Preparation for dying

Not all families are able to talk openly about the impending death, and sometimes parents or siblings are overwhelmed by grief. In other families there is quite open discussion between affected older children or adults and the family, and they have been able to bid farewell to family, friends and members of the CF team. When death seems inevitable, a decision by the patient and/or parents is required as to whether it would be better for this to occur at home or in hospital. When home is chosen, a key worker from the CF team, often the CF nurse, will act as the main link between the affected person, the family and the hospital. The aid of the general practitioner will generally be sought, and with the CF nurse arrangements are made for the dying person to be kept as comfortable as possible, with sedation where necessary. Some parents and relatives have found bereavement support groups helpful, others have found most comfort through their religion. The clinical psychologist can provide bereavement counselling where appropriate.

The parents and siblings

Cystic fibrosis may impose extra strains on the marriage, though some couples are drawn closer by it. The divorce rate is not higher amongst parents of a CF child than in the general population.

Healthy siblings may experience a number of difficulties. They may feel that they receive disproportionately less of their parents' time and thus feel neglected and resentful, with guilt feelings about their feelings of resentment. As they grow up, they may worry about their chances of being a carrier and their risk of having affected offspring themselves.

The mother: Mothers often carry the main burden of responsibility for treatment, with its taxing, daily demands. Of all the family members, including the affected person, mothers have been shown to have the greatest amount of knowledge about CF. They are also the most likely to become depressed from time to time. The depression is usually not so severe that they are unable to attend to all the demands of treatment. Rather it manifests as 'feeling blue' or being tired. If the mother herself is ill the family may need a great deal of support.

The father: On the whole, fathers involve themselves in the health and welfare of the child and in carrying out some of the treatment, especially physiotherapy. Where the father is the major breadwinner, this may limit his involvement and he may seldom be able to attend the CF clinic with his child. It may become habit for the father to opt out of assisting in the care of the affected child. Having an ill child may limit the family's earning capacity—it is difficult for both the mother and father to work, and choice of work or mobility are limited by the medical needs of the child. In countries where there is no national health service, the financial burdens of caring for a child or children with CF may be crippling.

Genetic aspects

The recent genetic discoveries have been hailed as great breakthroughs. Nevertheless, affected people have been heard to say that, thus far, no affected person's illness has been helped as a result of these discoveries. Prenatal diagnosis and termination of pregnancy pose a dilemma, especially for a condition affecting one's beloved child and for which treatment, no matter how burdensome, is available. On the other hand, couples may not wish to 'inflict' the condition on another child and may fear being left childless, should the affected child die; and there is their wish to have a healthy child. When a decision is made after careful thought and counselling to opt for prenatal testing, there may be heightened anxiety associated with the chorionic villus biopsy, the waiting for the results, the one in four who are told that the fetus is affected and who have to decide on whether to continue with the pregnancy or to have a termination. The couples' experiences during earlier prenatal tests and whether they resulted in termination may affect their decision. Couples who have had a termination do not get over the experience easily, though there is some evidence suggesting that the earlier in pregnancy a termination occurs, the less the long-term psychological effects.

Religious convictions may help some couples in their decisions, whilst others may feel pressured by their religion.

The genetic counselling team provides the parents with full support, whatever they decide to do. This is likely to minimize any possible psychological difficulties arising from the responsible decisions of informed couples.

Professional help

When psychological problems are prominent, there is generally one member of the CF team to whom the patient or parents best relate and through whom any modifications can be suggested. By virtue of his or her training, the clinical psychologist is best equipped to deal with particularly difficult or entrenched problems. Sometimes, the psychologist will decide to work through one of the other team members, when that seems best for the patient or family.

Conclusions

All the psychological problems which may occur in CF are functions of the particular circumstances that surround that family. None are really specific to CF. These problems may change, as new treatments with different demands are introduced.

6

Genetics of cystic fibrosis

INTRODUCTION: MITOSIS AND MEIOSIS

The human body is made up of a huge number of individual functional units called cells. These cells are too small to be seen by the naked eye, but they can be looked at through a microscope in which they are magnified maybe fifty to one hundred times. Each cell is surrounded by an outer membrane, within which are a number of structures essential to the working of the cell. The nucleus is one of these. It is surrounded by another membrane, and contains among other things the genetic information of the cell. All the cells of an individual have the same genetic information. It is this information that is responsible for the inherited characteristics of an individual.

Body cells are continually dividing during life; in this way the body can grow and repair itself. When a cell divides, it produces two daughter cells, each of which contains the same genetic information as the parent cell. To achieve this, the parental cell genetic information is duplicated before cell division so that there are two sets of this information, one for each daughter cell. This type of cell division is known as *mitosis*.

When the cell is not dividing, the genetic material is spread throughout the nucleus. However, when the cell is about to divide, the genetic material contracts and coils up. As a result of these changes, the structures in each cell that contain the genetic material (known as *chromosomes*) can be seen much more clearly as specific structural bodies (see Fig. 12). Chromosomes are asymmetrical structures consisting of a short (p) arm and a long (q) arm separated by a central constriction, the centrometre.

Different species have different numbers of chromosomes. Humans normally have forty-six chromosomes in all the cells of their body apart from the sex cells (the eggs or the sperm). Each of these body cells is *diploid*, i.e. it carries two complete sets of genetic information. Thus the forty-six chromosomes consist of two sets of twenty-three. One chromosome set comes from the mother via the ovum (egg) and the other comes from the father via the particular sperm that fertilized the ovum. Both

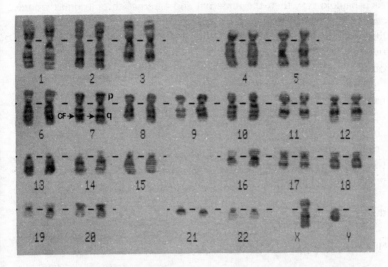

Fig. 12. The chromosomes of a normal human male individual. The banding pattern, produced with a specific stain, is characteristic of each pair of chromosomes. The CF gene is located half way down the long (q) arm of chromosome 7.

ovum and sperm are *haploid*, that is they carry only a single set of twenty-three chromosomes. When egg and sperm fuse in fertilization, the chromosome complement of the ensuing embryo is restored to forty-six (twenty-three pairs).

In twenty-two of these twenty-three pairs of chromosomes, members of the pair are the same in men and women. These pairs are known as the *autosomes*. The twenty-third pair comprises the sex chromosomes, X and Y. Normal women have two X chromosomes, normal men have one X chromosome and one Y. Unlike the autosome pairs, the X and Y chromosomes are functionally dissimilar. The Y chromosome is very small in comparison with the X and apparently carries very little genetic information, apart from that required to direct male sexual development.

As has already been mentioned, the ovum and the sperm only carry a single set of chromosomes. Eggs and sperm are made by a process called *meiosis*, a normal diploid cell with forty-six chromosomes divides into haploid cells containing twenty-three chromosomes each.

If meiosis simply involved one chromosome from each pair going into each haploid cell, then the maternal and paternal chromosomes would remain unchanged from generation to generation and there would be little genetic diversity. What actually happens is that during meiosis the two sets of genetic information in the cell are shuffled like two packs of cards. This process is known as recombination.

Before the cell divides in meiosis, the chromosomes join in homologous pairs. This means that chromosome 1 inherited from the mother joins up with the corresponding paternal chromosome, and likewise chromosome 2, 3, 4 etc. pair up. Random and reciprocal exchanges of genetic material then occur within each homologous pair, involving sections of genetic material from one chromosome breaking off and replacing the equivalent section on the other chromosome (see Fig. 13).

The two main chemical components of chromosomes are deoxyribonucleic acid (DNA) and proteins. It is the DNA that in its structure contains all the information needed to construct a human being from a single fertilized egg. The building blocks of DNA are chemical units of a

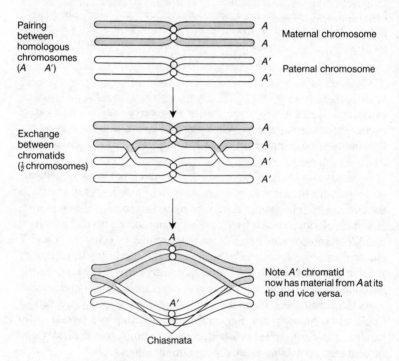

Fig. 13. Diagram to show recombination at meiosis.

base (a nitrogen containing compound, either a purine or a pyrimidine) and a sugar molecule (deoxyribose) joined together. Many of these units are linked through phosphate molecules into a long chain (see Fig. 14(a)). The four different bases that are used in DNA are called adenine (A), guanine (G), cytosine (C), and thymine (T). These are the elements of the genetic code (the 'language' of the genetic information). The DNA in chromosomes is in the form of a double chain, the so-called 'double helix', in which the two chains are wound round each other and joined together by their base units (see Fig. 14(b)). The structure can be likened to a spiral staircase where the two continuous sides (sugar–phosphate back bones) are joined at regular intervals by the stairs (bases) (see Fig. 14(c)). Due to differences in the sizes of the individual base molecules (adenine and guanine are bigger than cytosine and thymine), adenine can only join to thymine and guanine can only join to cytosine if the two sides of the staircase are to remain a constant distance apart.

Each DNA molecule can replicate itself, making an identical copy of its genetic information. This is what happens before mitosis, the cell division process described earlier. However, for this genetic information to be useful to the cell, it must be translated into a form that can be used by the cell machinery outside the nucleus. To achieve this the DNA has to be copied, or transcribed into another molecule, ribonucleic acid (RNA), otherwise known as messenger RNA. In turn, this messenger RNA is used as a blueprint for the translation of the genetic message into biologically useful molecules, proteins. Proteins are made up of a long chain of building blocks, called amino acids, that are joined together to form a functional whole. The base sequence in the RNA copy of the DNA directs the insertion of a particular amino acid in a specific place in each protein. Each amino acid corresponds to a set of three bases occurring in the RNA, and the nature of these three base coding units and the particular amino acids they correspond to, is called the genetic code. For example, a run of three adjacent bases TTT in the DNA would result in insertion of an amino acid called phenylalanine at that point in the particular protein chain being made. Many thousands of different proteins are made in the one cell. Proteins can really be regarded as the primary product of genetic information and all the different proteins made in an individual are responsible for his or her uniqueness. They have a wide range of functions in the body: structural proteins are major components of muscle, skin, hair and many other tissues, while enzymes are essential parts of the body's metabolic machinery.

Since all the cells in the body arise from mitotic division of the fertilized

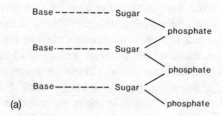

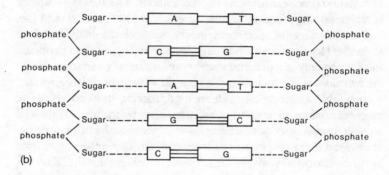

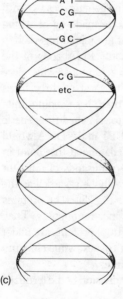

Fig. 14. The structure of DNA.
(a) The basic DNA chain
(b) Two DNA chains joined in a functional unit
(c) The double helix in three dimensions.

egg, each cell carries a full complement of genetic information, i.e. 46 chromosomes. However, only a very small part of this information is being used in any one cell at any one time. In fact, much of the DNA in the chromosomes never seems to be used at all in coding for proteins. The important coding regions of the DNA are found within functional units called *genes*. It is the coding regions within the genes that are transcribed into messenger RNA which then goes on to be the blueprint for protein manufacture, as we described above. Within and between genes or groups of genes are large non-coding regions of DNA. Some of these non-coding regions may have some role in controlling the activities of the genes, but the vast majority seem to have no function at all.

The cells of a particular tissue or organ will have a specific set of genes in action. Hence, though the enzyme-secreting cells of the pancreas and the cells lining the respiratory system will have certain active genes in common, (that is those making products that are essential for the maintenance of any living cell), other active genes will be coding for products involved in tissue-specific functions. For example, the pancreas secretory cells will have active genes producing specific digestive enzymes to break down food, while genes coding for mucus will be switched on in many of the cells lining the respiratory tract.

It should be remembered here that each cell contains a pair of each gene, one from each parent. Genes coding for the same product can vary slightly in their precise DNA sequence from one person to the next. Where an individual has inherited identical forms (alleles) of a particular gene from both parents he is said to be *homozygous* for that gene, but if he has inherited non-identical alleles for any specific gene he is defined as *heterozygous* for that gene. The words *heterozygote* and *carrier* of a particular gene are in some cases interchangeable.

Genetic diseases are caused by abnormal genes that do not fulfil their proper function. An abnormal gene can be classed as dominant or recessive. If an abnormal gene is dominant, its abnormality is manifest even if the other gene of the pair is normal. However, when an abnormal gene is recessive, the abnormality is masked if the other gene of the pair is normal. So a person who has CF or a similar recessive hereditary disease must be homozygous for the abnormal gene, i.e. they must have inherited the abnormal gene from both parents. An individual who is heterozygous (i.e. has one normal and one abnormal gene) for a recessive hereditary disease is known as a carrier of the abnormal gene. Carriers do not have the symptoms of the disease, but may pass it on to their offspring.

The combination of all the different genes that an individual has are known as his or her genotype. Simple inheritance patterns of dominant and recessive genes are illustrated in Fig. 15.

Both dominant and recessive diseases can be subdivided into autosomal and sex-linked conditions, which are coded for by genes located on the autosomes or on the sex chromosomes, respectively. The known inheritance pattern of the CF gene, derived from the study of many affected families, shows that equal numbers of male and female CF children are born to healthy parents. From this pattern it is clear that the CF gene must be autosomal and not sex-linked. Recessive diseases coded for by a gene on the X chromosome, such as haemophilia, are much more common in males than in females. This is because a male has only one X chromosome and so there is no possibility of a normal gene masking the defective one. For a female to be affected she would have to carry the same defect on both her X chromosomes, necessarily a rare event.

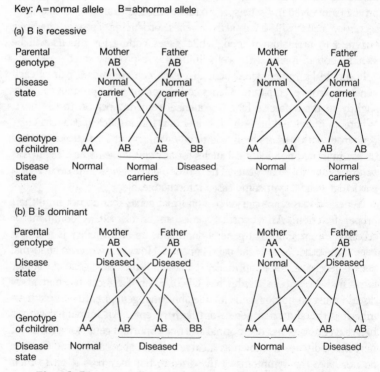

Fig. 15. Diagram to illustrate dominant and recessive inheritance.

Cystic fibrosis is an autosomal recessive disease, i.e. affected individuals inherit a defective gene from both parents. We have known since 1985 that the CF gene is located on the long (q) arm of chromosome 7 (see Fig. 12). However, there is no visible abnormality in chromosome structure; the fault is a much more subtle change within the DNA molecule. The classical inheritance pattern of the CF gene from two carrier parents is shown in Fig. 16.

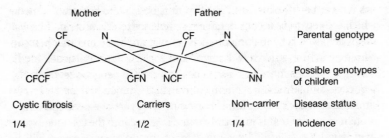

Fig. 16. Inheritance of the CF gene from two carrier parents. CF = CF gene, N = normal gene.

THE CYSTIC FIBROSIS GENE

Discovery

In the autumn of 1989, it was announced by collaborating research groups in Toronto, Canada, and Michigan, America, that the cystic fibrosis gene had been isolated. This had been the ultimate goal of an enormous research effort that had been going on in several laboratories in North America, Canada, and Britain for nearly ten years.

However, isolation of the CF gene is by no means the end of the story. In many ways it marks the beginning of our understanding of how the disease of cystic fibrosis actually happens. With the CF gene in hand, researchers can now start to ask the fundamental biological questions about the disease. In other words, how does the CF gene make an individual's lungs become blocked with mucus secretions and susceptible to recurrent infections; why does CF cause the pancreatic ducts to become blocked with mucus secretions; how does the CF gene cause sweat to be too salty and why does it cause sterility in most men with CF? It is only through these questions being answered that more effective treatments for CF will become possible.

What is the CF gene and what protein does it code for?

At the time of writing we cannot yet answer this fundamental question. However, we do know that the gene is very large in terms of the amount of DNA it contains and we know the base sequence of the important coding regions within the gene (see p. 75). From this DNA sequence information we can predict the type of protein that the gene is likely to code for. In other words, though the protein produced from the CF gene has not yet been isolated and purified, it is possible to construct a model which is likely to bear considerable resemblance to this protein. The way this is achieved is by making predictions that are based on other proteins whose structure is already known, and looking for similarities in the coding DNA sequence in these genes and the CF gene sequence. DNA sequence similarities are often equivalent to functional or structural similarities at the protein level. For example, if part of a gene codes for a protein sequence that is invariably found inserted into the cell membrane, then it is likely that at least this part of the unknown protein will be anchored to the cell membrane.

On the basis of such structure predictions, it appears that the protein encoded by the CF gene is probably located in the membrane surrounding cells or in an internal membrane and that it has some role in policing the entry or exit of some as yet undefined substance from that cell.

Where is the CF gene active?

We have already discussed the fact that not all the genetic information is used in each specialized cell type in the body (p. 75). The cystic fibrosis gene is likely to be active in cells or tissues that are directly affected by the disease process. Cells within the lungs and respiratory system, the pancreas and digestive system, the sweat gland and the male genital ducts. In particular, the CF gene must be important in the highly specialized cells (epithelial cells) that line the duct systems of all these organs. The specialized epithelia where the CF protein is functionally important, include the sheets of cells lining the lungs, the pancreatic ducts, the male genital ducts, the sweat gland duct, and possibly other systems.

What do these specialized epithelial cells have in common? The most important common characteristic, at least with respect to their malfunctioning in CF, is that they all secrete substances into the lumen of the duct they line. In the lung, pancreatic duct, and male genital duct, the substances are mainly mucus secretions in a salt solution. In the sweat gland duct only a salt solution is produced. The exact type of salt and of mucus secreted varies from one duct lining to another. For example, the sweat gland duct secretes mainly sodium chloride (common salt) while the pancreatic duct lining produces a bicarbonate solution which is important for maintaining the right pH (level of acidity; see p. 20) for pancreatic enzymes to work properly in the duodenum. Based on what we already know about the probable structure of the CF protein, as predicted from its DNA sequence, we can speculate on where and how it operates. It seems likely that the protein will be located in or close to the surface membrane or an internal membrane of the specialized ductal epithelial cells that we have talked about. From the vantage point of the surface membrane the CF protein would be well-placed to regulate the movements of salt molecules out of the epithelial cells and into the duct lumen, or vice versa. Hence, the CF gene product has been called the cystic fibrosis transmembrane conductance regulator (CFTR). Indeed, there is already ample evidence from measurements carried out in the laboratory on small pieces of sweat gland duct and lung epithelium, that in CF the movements of salts (charged ions; hence the name conductance regulator) across these epithelia are not properly controlled. How exactly this abnormal regulation of salt movements happens in CF is still not known. It is still quite possible that the CF gene itself only indirectly causes abnormal regulation of salt movements and that its primary function is quite different. For example, it might affect secretion of an un-related substance. However, now the CF gene has been isolated, research scientists are beginning to have the tools they need in order to sort out this complex question. It is likely that it will be necessary to find out how the protein made by the non-defective counterpart of the CF gene works before we can fully understand what the CF defect does to the protein.

What are the mutations in the CF gene that cause the disease?

A gene the size of the CF gene contains an enormous amount of genetic information in terms of physical amounts of DNA. An abnormality in any part of that DNA could result in the CF gene product being defective. In other words, remembering that genetic information is stored in DNA which is transcribed into a messenger RNA intermediate, which in turn is translated into a functional protein, many different defects at the DNA level can cause the same protein to be defective. Of course, the precise defect at the DNA level will correspond to a specific abnormality in the protein but all defects in the same protein are likely, in general, to cause the same disease. In this way, the disease cystic fibrosis could be caused by a whole range of different lesions (mutations) at the DNA level. As it turns out, in northern European and North American populations, about 70 per cent of CF mutated genes carry exactly the same lesion. That lesion is the loss of three bases in the DNA sequence of the CF gene, which translates into the loss of one amino acid in the protein that is coded for by the CF gene (see p. 73). This amino acid is the phenyl-alanine (F) found at amino acid position 508 in the CFTR protein, and so the common mutation is referred to as the delta F508 deletion. In southern European populations the frequency of this mutation is much lower, somewhere in the order of 30–50 per cent of CF genes having this defect. When it was discovered, late in 1989 that 70 per cent of North American and northern European CF genes carried the same defect, it was hoped that maybe there might be a relatively small number of other lesions that accounted for all the other defective CF genes. That would have made population screening for the CF gene an imminent possibility (see Genetic screening section, p. 91). However, by the Autumn of 1990 it was already clear that there were more than 60 other lesions in the CF gene DNA that could cause the same disease. Most of these seemed to cause CF in only one or a relatively small number of patients, which makes the idea of population screening infinitely more complex.

FREQUENCY OF CF

As has already been mentioned, CF is the most common potentially lethal autosomal recessive disease among Caucasians (white Indo-Europeans). The condition is excessively rare among Chinese races and in African Negroes. CF does occur in black Americans, natives of many Middle Eastern countries, and in Pakistan. In Caucasian races, however, the CF carrier frequency is about one in 22 to 25 individuals, and one baby in around 2000 to 2500 live births has the disease.

How can we explain the high frequency of CF if 98 per cent of adult males with the disorder are sterile, and until very recently females with CF were not growing up to have children?

(a) Heterozygote advantage

Many doctors and scientists believe that the high CF gene frequency is due to some heterozygote advantage. That is, carriers of the CF gene (those with one CF gene and one normal gene) have a higher reproductive input into the population than non-carriers. This could be because more CF carriers reach child-producing age, or because CF carriers have more children than non-carriers. The overall effect is that the CF gene is reintroduced into the population in each generation at a slightly higher frequency than its normal counterpart. Heterozygote advantage is still only a theory, i.e. it has not been proved. Explanations of the causes of heterozygote advantage are generally based on the idea of increased resistance to other potentially lethal diseases. One such theoretical explanation is given below.

Cholera

One possible theory to account for CF heterozygote advantage relates to the known abnormalities in the movement of salts (particularly chloride), in and out of certain body cells and tissues in CF (see above and Chapter 2, p. 26). It has been suggested that defective chloride ion transport might reduce the severity of cholera by inhibiting water loss from the intestine. Cholera is no longer an important disease in Western nations, but the CF gene frequency does not seem to be falling (although in genetic terms it may be too early for such a change to be obvious). Similar theories based on resistance to tuberculosis and influenza, do not seem very probable.

(b) Reproductive compensation

One further possibility to account for maintenance of an unusually high frequency for the CF gene, before reliable diagnosis of CF was possible, was reproductive compensation. This theory suggests that families where a child has CF generally have more children, to 'compensate' for the possible death of the affected child. Two out of three of the healthy children will be carriers of the CF gene (see p. 77, in this chapter), so more CF genes are introduced into the population. In most instances where this theory has been studied in the past, the mean size of families with a CF child has been larger than that of families with no CF children. However, it is unlikely that this reproductive compensation is a major factor at the present time.

(c) Consanguinity

Consanguinity is inbreeding between genetically related members of the same family (for example, brother and sister, first cousins or uncle and niece). In certain countries consanguinous marriages may play a part in increasing the incidence of what might otherwise be a rarer genetic condition (although consanguinity appears to have little effect in CF in most countries). In a few isolated communities, notably amongst Afrikaaners in Namibia, a much higher incidence of CF than expected has been found. In these instances the parents of those children affected could be traced back to common forebears, generations earlier. One genealogy of the Afrikaaner population in Namibia, drawn up by one of the authors (M.S.) when he worked there, is shown in Fig. 17.

RISK FACTORS

What are the chances of having a child with cystic fibrosis?

Until very recently the best that genetic counsellors could do in attempting to answer this question was refer to charts such as Tables 2 and 3 . These are mathematical calculations based on the frequency of the disease (1 in 2000 people) and the estimated frequency of the carrier state (1 in 22 individuals in the general population). If a couple has had a child with CF it is clear that they must both be carriers (heterozygous). In this case, the chance that any of their offspring will have CF (i.e. will be homozygous for the abnormal gene) will remain 1 in 4 for each pregnancy (see Fig. 16 on inheritance patterns of the CF gene). The healthy brother or sister of someone with CF has a 2 in 3 chance of being a CF carrier (one abnormal and one normal gene) and a 1 in 3 chance of not carrying a CF gene at all. Actual examples of the inheritance pattern of the CF gene are shown in the family trees of Fig. 18.

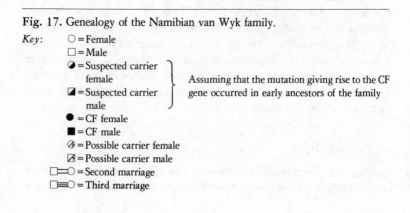

Fig. 17. Genealogy of the Namibian van Wyk family.

Key: ○ = Female
        □ = Male
        ◖ = Suspected carrier ⎫
            female   ⎪ Assuming that the mutation giving rise to the CF
        ◪ = Suspected carrier ⎬ gene occurred in early ancestors of the family
            male   ⎭
        ● = CF female
        ■ = CF male
        ⊘ = Possible carrier female
        ◪ = Possible carrier male
        □━○ = Second marriage
        □≡○ = Third marriage

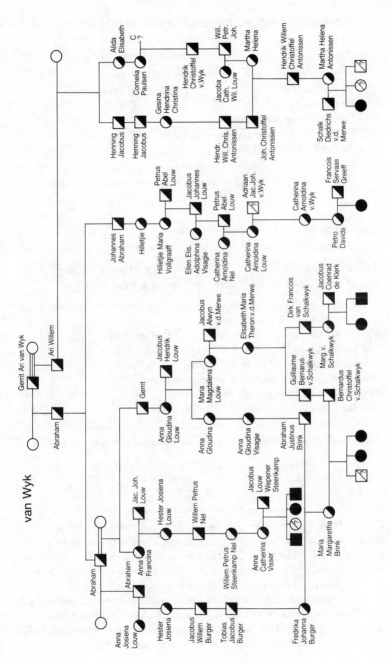

Table 2. Chances of being a CF carrier

History	Chance
Mother has CF[a]	1/1 (i.e. definite)
Brother or sister has CF	2/3
Half-brother or sister has CF	1/2
Brother or sister has offspring with CF	1/2
No family history of CF	1/22

[a] Males with CF are generally sterile and so are not inlcuded in the table.

Table 3. Risks of having a child with CF (based on an assumption that one in twenty-two of the general population are carriers)

Couples with one or more CF children	1/4
Mother has CF[a]: partner has no history of CF in the family	1/44
One parent has had a child with CF: partner has no history	1/88
Brother or sister of child with CF: partner has no history	1/132
Brother or sister of parent of CF child: partner has no history	1/176
First cousins: no history of CF in the family	1/700
Unrelated couples: no history of CF in the family	1/2000

[a] Males with CF are generally sterile and so are not included in the above table.

Fig. 18. Some illustrative family pedigrees. If one analysed a sufficient number of families and made allowances for those instances where both parents are carriers yet none of their children has CF, then the results would show that, where both parents are carriers, one in four of their children will be born with CF. More or less equal numbers of males and females are born with CF.

The numbers in the diagram indicate the ages of CF patients and their brothers and sisters at the time of writing, or the ages at which CF patients died (4/12 denotes four months). The chances of each non-affected brother or sister of a CF child being a CF carrier are referred to in Table 2.

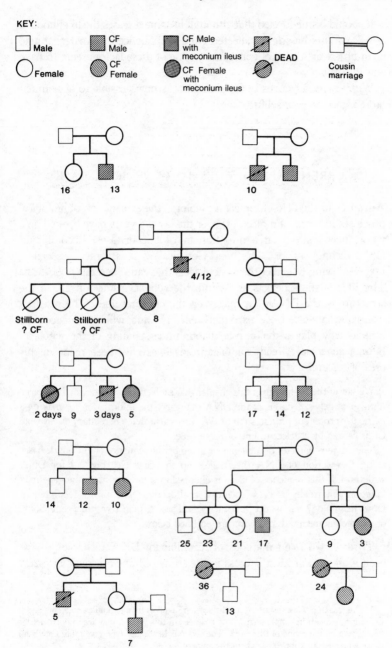

It should be mentioned that although in some diseases the likelihood of at-risk parents having an affected child is influenced by maternal age, birth order, or season of conception, none of these factors seem to have any role in CF.

With recent advances in CF genetics it is now possible to offer much more informed counselling.

CURRENT APPROACHES TO GENETIC DISEASE[a]

Advances in the field of molecular biology (the explanation of biological processes in terms of molecules) over the last 15 years have opened up a whole new research area into human genetic diseases. Recombinant DNA technology, or 'The New Genetics' as it is sometimes called, involves trying to detect the basic defects that cause hereditary diseases. The sites of these defects are within the genetic material itself, in the structure of the DNA that makes up the chromosomes. The research techniques involved are extremely effective and will, in due course, undoubtedly play a major role in our understanding of the whole of human genetics. Already significant advances have been made in this area of research.

We saw at the beginning of this chapter that each chromosome contains a large number of genes, sections of the DNA that carry the information for making a particular protein or protein subunit. We also learnt that a hereditary disease like CF is caused by a defect in one of these genes.

The unique character of each gene is given by the sequence of nucleotide bases along the section of DNA that makes up the gene (see Fig. 14 for DNA structure). If this sequence of bases is changed in some way, then the gene may function abnormally or cease to function altogether. The aim of recombinant DNA technology is to detect these changes of base sequence within a gene. Some of the techniques used to do this are outlined below.

To date two main methods of recombinant DNA technology have been used with greatest success in the study of human genetic diseases.

---

[a] The research work discussed in this section involves many complex concepts and is difficult to explain in simple terms. The passages in this section that are in normal-sized type give a basic outline of this work. The sections in smaller type give more details for those who wish to know more about the subject.

One involves indirect analysis of the gene concerned. This is achieved by studying a known piece of DNA that is physically and genetically linked to the disease gene. (If two genes are located on the same stretch of DNA sufficiently close to each other, then the study of the behaviour of one gene at cell division may provide information on the likely behaviour of the other.) The other method of genetic analysis concerns the direct study of the disease gene itself.

Indirect analysis of a gene

At various locations throughout the human genetic material (the genome) there exist what are known as polymorphic sites. The sequence of bases on the DNA at these sites varies from individual to individual. These polymorphisms can be detected within the total cellular DNA by the use of DNA 'probe' molecules specific for each polymorphism. Polymorphic sites thus make good 'markers' within the genetic material. They occur sufficiently frequently for there to exist several by chance within close proximity to any gene coding for a hereditary disease. These genetic markers can be used to indirectly study and locate genes that code for hereditary diseases.

The polymorphic sites can be detected by a class of enzymes called restriction endonucleases. These enzymes recognize particular combinations of nucleotide sequence within the DNA and cleave the DNA at their 'recognition sites'. If the nucleotide sequence at one of these 'recognition sites' is altered the enzyme will no longer recognize it and so the DNA will not be cut. This natural variation in nucleotide sequence has thus caused a 'restriction fragment length polymorphism' (RFLP) since it has caused one restriction endonuclease to produce different length DNA fragments in different people. The DNA probes that are used to identify RFLPs in the living cell are segments of DNA that are complementary (i.e. will combine with) all or part of the DNA sequence of interest.

It is likely that any human gene will have, somewhere in the neighbouring DNA, one or more of these polymorphic markers. If a marker is closely linked to a particular gene in physical terms (that is, in terms of linear distance along the DNA molecule) then it is probable that at each generation the gene concerned and the marker will be inherited together. If a marker is not close to the particular gene on the chromosome, then when gametes (eggs or sperm) are formed by meiosis, the marker and the gene may become separated during recombination (see p. 72). The closer a marker is to the gene of interest, the more likely it is that gene and marker will remain linked over several generations.

Using the probes (mentioned above) for polymorphic markers, it is possible to look for linkage between a marker and the gene for a particular disease, even when the precise location of the gene is not known. Researchers will try probes for many markers, and look for their recurrence over several generations in a family that is know to carry the gene for the disease of interest. By chance a linkage may be found between the abnormal gene and one or more polymorphic markers. That is, within any one family all individuals who have the disease will have one form of the polymorphism while all those who are unaffected will have the other form. In the case of a recessive disease carriers will have both forms of the polymorphism.

Once a link between the disease gene and a marker has been found, that marker can be used in a variety of ways. First, it can be used in genetic counselling and prenatal diagnosis, even if the gene has not been identified. Second, it can sometimes be used to find out which individuals in a family are carriers of a defective gene (see Fig. 19). Linked markers may also remain useful in family studies even when a disease gene has

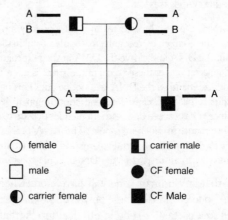

Fig. 19. Use of linked DNA markers to follow the inheritance of CF genes. A and B are two forms of a probe very closely linked to the CF gene. The two CF carrier parents each have band A and band B; one unaffected child only has band B while the affected child only has band A. Thus each parent carries their CF gene on their chromosome carrying band A and the normal counterpart on the chromosome carrying band B. The unaffected child who has both bands A and B is a CF carrier.

been isolated, in particular,when the precise defect in the gene has not been pin-pointed in a particular family.

The use of markers linked to the CF gene

Since the end of 1985, DNA markers linked to the CF gene have been available. The first set of markers were reasonably far, in physical terms, from the CF gene itself. As a result there was still an unacceptably high chance that the marker and the CF gene could become separated during egg and sperm formation, so causing errors in diagnosis. This first set of markers rapidly paved the way for the isolation of DNA markers that were substantially nearer to the gene.

Each polymorphic marker probe linked to the CF gene may be used in tests that can be carried out on DNA derived from any tissue as well as from blood cells. For example, in a prenatal test, cells from the chorionic villi or from amniotic fluid may be used (see p. 92). The total DNA in these cells, including that from chromosome 7 (which carries the CF gene) is digested into small pieces using certain specific enzymes and tested with the probes.

The chemical reactions that occur give rise to specific patterns of bands corresponding to pieces of DNA of different sizes. These band patterns can then be compared in the person with CF, his or her parents, brothers and sisters, or with the patterns of an unborn child in the same family.

The example illustrated in Fig. 19 shows a sample test result.

As has already been mentioned, because one is not dealing with the CF gene itself in these indirect tests, but with linked DNA marker probes, there is a built-in error rate. This rate depends on the frequency with which the linked probe is separated from the CF gene during egg and sperm formation. This major disadvantage of indirect tests is circumvented when one can directly analyse a disease gene rather than using linked markers to track it from one generation to the next.

Direct analysis of a gene

As has already been discussed, the CF gene was isolated in the autumn of 1989. This has opened up a completely new degree of accuracy in genetic counselling for the disease. Scientists can now look directly at the DNA in the CF gene in different individuals to search for defects. We know that about 70 per cent of people carrying a defective CF gene in

England, northern European countries and North America, all have the same lesion in their DNA. Three bases (see p. 80) are absent from the middle of their CF gene, which results in the loss of one amino acid building block from the protein that is coded for by the CF gene. The loss of these three bases can be easily detected by a rather simple test.

DNA is extracted from the blood cells of an individual, and the specific region of DNA containing the CF gene is amplified many hundreds of times. The amplification involves using an enzyme to synthesize many identical copies of that individual's DNA between specified points on either side of the missing three base-pairs. For example, if those specified points are particular DNA sequences that are 50 bases apart in normal individuals, the same specified points would only be 47 bases apart in CF individuals with the common lesion.

This change can readily be seen when the amplified DNA fragments are separated on the basis of their size (Fig. 20).

Figure 20 shows a 50 (normal gene) or 47 (CF gene) base-pair DNA fragment amplified from the CF gene of two CF carrier parents, their unaffected non-carrier child, and their affected child. The parents each have one 47 and one 50 base-pair fragment corresponding to their CF and normal genes respectively. The unaffected non-carrier child has two copies of the 50 base-pair normal fragment. The affected child has two copies of the 47 base-pair CF fragment only.

This simple test can not only be used in tracking the CF gene in families known to be carrying CF genes that have the common mutation. It is equally valid as a carrier screening test in the general population. However, here again, it will only detect about 70 per cent of CF carriers since the other 30 per cent will have other defects in their CF gene that will require alternative tests. These tests will be similar to the one

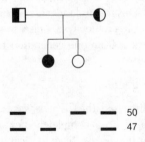

Fig. 20. Detection of the three base-pair deletion that causes CF in 70 per cent of defective CF genes. (See Key to Fig. 19.)

described for the common CF mutation, but they will amplify different parts of the CF gene specific to each different mutation.

Until all the mutations in the CF gene have been defined, it is a matter of debate whether to offer general carrier screening for the whole population, since not all CF genes will be detected. If it turns out that the 30 per cent of the CF genes in the population that do not have the common three base-pair deletion, have one of a relatively small number of other mutations, then it will be relatively simple to offer population screening with a small number of diagnostic tests. However, if it turns out that there are hundreds of possible mutations in the CF gene then it will be rather difficult to have an efficient population screening programme. To date (October 1990) more than 60 rare mutations have been found in the CF gene, and many of these have only been found in one affected individual. Unless a few more common mutations are found soon it is likely that generalized CF population screening will be greatly delayed. However, with a disease as common as CF (1 in 22 people being carriers), some sort of screening programme is likely to be developed even if it cannot pick up all carriers.

Once two potential parents are known to be carriers of CF, either due to the previous birth of an affected child or following direct genetic testing, they can be offered prenatal diagosis of CF at future pregnancies.

METHODS OF PRENATAL DIAGNOSIS

The methods described below are currently used to diagnose a number of diseases before birth. Most methods of prenatal diagnosis rely on obtaining a small sample of material from, or produced by, the unborn child (the fetus). A biochemical test or a study of the chromosomes can then be carried out on this sample. This material may be a sample of amniotic fluid (the fluid surrounding the developing embryo, which contains many cell types that have been shed by the fetus and the membranes around it), a sample of the fetal blood taken from the umbilical cord or a small piece of the rumpled outer surface of the membranes surrounding the fetus, known as chorionic villi (see Fig. 21). All the procedures discussed have an acceptably low risk of interfering with the pregnancy, and have been used successfully in the prenatal diagnosis of a variety of different genetic diseases.

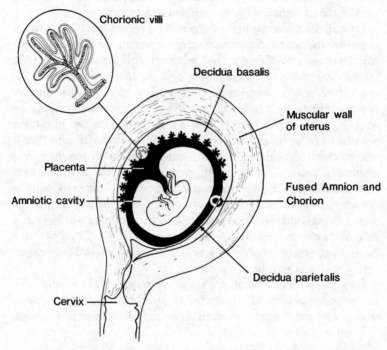

Fig. 21. Diagram to show the human embryo in the amniotic sac about twelve weeks into the pregnancy.

Amniocentesis

This test is usually carried out 16 to 18 weeks into the pregnancy. It involves collecting a small amount of amniotic fluid from around the fetus. It was the first technique developed for prenatal diagnosis of fetal abnormalities and is still the most frequently used. Following amniocentesis there is slightly less than one per cent increase in the chance of a miscarriage, and around a one per cent increase in the chance of a premature birth. Several tests can be carried out on this amniotic fluid. The fluid itself may have certain biochemical measurements carried out on it directly. For example, the level of a particular protein called alpha-fetoprotein that is present in amniotic fluid is characteristically found to be higher in defects of spine development such as spina bifida. There are also cells present in the amniotic fluid, and these may be grown (cultured) in the laboratory. The cultured cells can then be analysed to look for markers that are characteristic of particular diseases. One such marker is the number of chromosomes within each cell. Fetuses that have Down's syndrome (commonly known as mongolism), for example, carry three copies of chromosome 21 instead of the usual two.

Fetal blood sampling

This more recent technique involves taking a blood sample from the unborn child. The blood is most readily drawn from the vessels in the umbilical cord. The method has been used successfully in the prenatal diagnosis of thalassaemias (defects in the structure of haemoglobin, the molecule that carries oxygen around the blood system). The test is performed after about 18 weeks of pregnancy. It carries a small (1 per cent) risk of miscarriage.

Chorionic villus sampling

Amniocentesis and fetal blood sampling are only useful for diagnosis at a quite late stage of pregnancy (16 to 18 weeks). At such a late stage, termination of the pregnancy is very difficult for the mother, both physically and mentally. Chorionic villus sampling, however, can be carried out much earlier in the pregnancy (between 8 and 12 weeks after conception). The method involves the physical removal of a small piece of the rumpled outer surface (villi) of the membranes surrounding the fetus (the chorion). (Part of the chorion forms the placenta later in pregnancy: see Fig. 21.) Rapid results can be obtained with chorionic villus sampling, because tests are carried out directly on the sample itself. This is in contrast to amniocentesis, where cells from the amniotic fluid must be grown in the laboratory until enough cells have been produced for testing. Hence chorionic villus sampling provides a method of early diagnosis of hereditary disorders. The risk factors associated with this procedure are nearly as low as those for amniocentesis. Allowing for the natural loss of about 4 per cent of fetuses between around 10 weeks gestation and normal term, chorionic villus sampling increases this figure to around 6 per cent (in other words an added 2 per cent risk).

The basis of the procedure is to locate the position of the developing fetus and the chorionic tissue using ultrasound (see Fig. 21). Solid objects deflect very high frequency sound waves (ultrasound) passed across the abdomen and these deflections are translated into an image of the developing pregnancy on a television screen. A thin, hollow tube is then passed through the cervix (the neck of the womb) and guided to the chorion using the image on the ultrasound scan. A very small piece of chorion (about 2 mm wide) is sucked into the tube and removed for testing. The sample may also be taken through the wall of the abdomen, similar to amniocentesis. Chorion tissue is growing very rapidly at this stage in pregnancy, so the cells in the sample will be dividing fast. This is ideal for rapid chromosome analysis, as well as for direct investigation using the techniques of biochemistry and molecular biology. The vast majority of prenatal diagnostic tests for CF are now carried out by chorionic villus sampling (CVS).

Ultrasound

As explained in the previous section, ultrasound can be used to obtain a picture of the developing pregnancy. This image on its own can be useful in showing up certain abnormalities in the unborn child. These are generally malformations of the fetus that alter its normal appearance in an ultrasound scan; for example, large-scale abnormalities of the spinal cord. Meconium ileus, the blockage of the bowel that occurs in some CF babies and was discussed in Chapter 2, may occasionally be detected by ultrasound scanning. Its role in prenatal diagnosis is a very limited one, but it may be useful in conjunction with other tests in suggesting that a fetus may have CF. Ultrasound has the advantage of being non-invasive and so does not increase the chance of spontaneous miscarriage.

Pre-implantation testing for CF

It is likely that in the not too distant future it will be possible to detect a genetic disease such as CF in the fertilized embryo when it only contains a few cells and has not yet implanted into the womb. The test will involve using the technique that is already well-established in the treatment of infertility and is known as *in vitro* fertilization. This involves removing eggs from a woman and fertilizing them with her partner's sperm in a test-tube. The ensuing embryos are then placed back in the mother's womb to implant and develop into healthy babies. It is possible to remove one cell from the embryo at a very early stage and the fetus still develops perfectly normally. The DNA in the cell that has been removed can then be analysed directly using the amplification methods described above (p. 90). If the cell is found to have the CF lesion then that embryo will not be implanted into the mother, and further tests will be done to identify an embryo that does not have the disease. By this method, though it is at present still technically extremely difficult and unlikely to be generally available for some time, a future child can be shown not to have a specific genetic disease even prior to starting development as a fetus. Some couples would find this more acceptable than prenatal diagnosis and early abortion. This group includes those who have had prenatal diagnosis in the past, which may have resulted in the abortion of an affected fetus; those who by religious or moral conviction view pre-implantation diagnosis as different to antenatal diagnosis during pregnancy and couples who will not accept abortion.

Prenatal diagnostic tests for CF

It is now possible to offer the vast majority of couples at risk for CF a prenatal diagnostic test for the disease. The precise test offered, whether it is a direct analysis of the DNA within the CF gene or an indirect test using markers linked to the CF gene, will be a DNA-based test. In other words, the test will be carried out on DNA extracted from fetal tissue (be it chorionic villi or single cells) in the same way as tests are done on the DNA in the blood cells of the parents.

There is one exception to this DNA-based testing and that is a means of diagnosing CF that until quite recently had a specific role in enabling more couples to have a prenatal diagnostic test for the disease. The 'Brock test' was useful in at least two relatively frequent situations. The first of these was when the only CF child in a family had already died so it was not possible to establish which of each of the parental chromosome 7s carried a defective CF gene (before the CF gene was cloned and all diagnosis was being done on the basis of linked DNA markers). The second situation when the Brock test was invaluable was when a woman at high risk of having a CF child, as a result of her family history of previous children, did not reach the counselling clinic until it was too late to carry out a DNA-based test on chorionic villi. The latter test is not usually carried out after about 12 weeks of pregnancy.

The Brock test measures the levels of three specific proteins in the amniotic fluid surrounding the fetus. All three are substantially less abundant than normal in amniotic fluid from CF fetuses. Unfortunately, this test does produce between 5 and 10 per cent of incorrect results; that is, normal fetuses diagnosed as having CF and CF fetuses diagnosed as being normal. However, as more and more mutations in the CF gene are defined the role of this test gradually declines.

GENETIC COUNSELLING IN CF

Genetic counsellors in the UK are medically qualified and may or may not specialize in genetics. The paediatrician or physician at the CF clinic may provide the counselling. When a couple or individual ask for genetic counselling there is an inference that they would wish to know the answers to certain questions. In providing these answers the counsellor will need to provide an understanding of the disorder. In the case of CF, this will include the possible ranges of severity in different affected individuals; the burden of the condition both for the affected person and the family; the types and effectiveness of the life-long treatment necessary and a word on life-expectancy.

Parents of newly diagnosed children with CF may not know all the implications of the diagnosis and will need this information to help them to exercise their options. When the illness itself has been discussed the risks of recurrence in any further children born will be mentioned and the autosomal recessive nature of CF explained.

Parents whose children are born with meconium ileus and who turn out to have CF, are especially in need of counselling. We have seen that meconium ileus in newborn children is very often associated with subsequent CF affected babies also having meconium ileus. In two cases known to the authors, children were born with meconium ileus and had to be operated on, but by the age of eight months these babies were thriving. The parents of these children found the experience of their children being born with meconium ileus extremely traumatic, and felt that CF without meconium ileus would have been preferable to meconium ileus alone. The children are now aged 8 and 9 years respectively and neither set of young parents has added to the family, still quoting the meconium ileus as the main reason. They have not been encouraged by the availability of prenatal tests for the presence or absence of CF.

A risk of 1 in 4 of having another affected child, as it would be for parents of a child with CF, constitutes a high risk with the same chance of occurring as of two coins falling 'heads'. Couples who realize the magnitude of this risk may wish to discuss options open to them.

Before 1985, prenatal diagnosis for CF was not available and couples either decided to have no further children; to take the 1 in 4 risk; to adopt or to have artificial insemination using donor sperm (to reduce the odds of having an affected child). Occasionally, parents of a child with CF divorce and the genetic implications may have played a role in this since their risk with a new partner would be reduced.

Although some studies have shown the parents of children with CF to be less put off having further children than parents of children with other serious hereditary diseases, the general tendency has been for the child with CF to be the last born to that couple. For several disorders (for example, spina bifida or Down's syndrome) the existence of prenatal tests for these diseases has influenced couples and encouraged them to undertake a further pregnancy in the knowledge that the presence of the disorder can be excluded or confirmed in the unborn baby. They understand that they would opt for abortion if the disorder were to be diagnosed in the fetus. Before the existence of a test for CF, in an American study, parents who had children with CF were asked what they thought about the idea of a prenatal test to diagnose CF. The majority of parents said that they would be interested, though a number said they would not want such tests to be performed and others said they would not opt to end the pregnancy.

Of course, people differ very strongly in their views on abortion and prenatal diagnosis in general. For couples at risk of having a child with CF, the existence of real treatment possibilities and the good chances of the child reaching adulthood in reasonable health may be strong arguments against prenatal tests.

It is a sad fact that diagnosing CF prenatally would not help to cure the unborn child. Prenatal diagnosis of CF would only offer two options; abortion or birth of an affected child.

Until recently we were unable to diagnose CF prenatally so there was no option of prenatal diagnosis with abortion of the affected fetus. Now this has changed dramatically; first, with the discovery of the exact chromosomal position of the CF gene, and in many cases now with a test based on the exact genetic abnormality (see p. 80). These tests are sufficiently accurate for them to be offered prospectively. The genetic counselling session has become very factual and we are, except in extremely rare situations, able to differentiate the CF-bearing chromosome from the one free of a defective CF gene in both parents. This is achieved using tests based either on a change within the CF gene itself (see Fig. 20) or by analysing the inheritance of DNA that is physically very close to the CF gene (see Fig. 19). Thus we are able to predict with increasing accuracy if a fetus is destined to be affected with CF, a healthy carrier, or free of CF genes. Also, we are able to test healthy siblings of someone with CF to see if they are carriers or not (see later).

When couples opt to have prenatal testing for CF, this generally means tests on DNA obtained from chorionic villi (see p. 93) taken at 8–10 weeks of pregnancy. Most women are already 5–6 weeks pregnant when they first realize it. This means that couples need to inform the geneticist immediately, to allow time for the necessary clinical and laboratory arrangements to be made. The exact duration of pregnancy will be confirmed by ultrasound examination. Ideally, couples will have decided on this course of action *before* starting a pregnancy, and their genetic status and that of their affected child will already be known. This will enable the laboratory test that is relevant to their particular case to be run directly. If couples are referred for counselling for the first time while a pregnancy is already underway, tests for CF are still feasible, but the parent's decisions, based on laboratory results, will not be taken as coolly. Furthermore, extra laboratory time and expense is required when tests need to be undertaken urgently on top of the routine ones. When couples are referred after 11 or 12 weeks of pregnancy, one may still be able to offer CF testing at 15–16 weeks, following amniocentesis and analysis of fetal cells in the amniotic fluid. However, the late result will necessitate a mid-trimester abortion if the parents decide to terminate an affected fetus. Most tests for CF are now done using a DNA amplification technique (see p. 90) that allows rapid testing, so results are usually available within a day of running the relevant test.

As we have already discussed (see p. 80), in September 1989 the commonest abnormality *within* the CF gene was discovered. The incidence of this exact abnormality varies in different countries, but it comprises about 70 per cent of CF genes in the UK. Thus, a test based on this specific abnormality could detect 70 per cent of carriers, even in the absence of a family history. Put another way, a negative test result in such a person would reduce their risk to 30 per cent of 1 in 22 (this being the frequency of CF carriers in the general population); that is, 1 in 73. Anyone whose test is positive is established as a carrier, and this has very useful implications in genetic counselling. Several groups who often request genetic counselling now are: first, siblings of those with CF; second, siblings of the parents of a CF child who wish to be tested together with their spouses; third, new partners of a parent of a CF child. Even if the CF child has died, such testing may allow carrier status to be excluded or become much less likely. Further, distant relatives of a CF patient, aware of their increased risks of being carriers can have themselves tested with their partners. Cystic fibrosis carrier-state testing would also be wise for partners of women with CF who might want to undertake pregnancies, and for sperm donors when artificial insemination is undertaken by those with a family history of CF.

Since only 1 in 22 of the general population carries a CF gene, most testing of partners of those with a family history of CF gives negative results. Even if the person with the CF family history tests positive, the combined risk of having an affected child with a partner who tests negative is $1/73 \times 1/4 = 1/292$. This is generally taken as an encouraging figure by most of those tested and many undertake or continue with pregnancy. Of course, occasionally, testing shows both partners to be carriers and so at a 1/4 risk of having a CF child. Then all the options open to parents of affected children become available.

Many laboratories have joined in an international consortium to discover the remaining 30 per cent of abnormalities in the CF gene. When the majority of these have been pin-pointed, general population screening of those at or approaching reproductive age will become possible. Early pilot studies of population screening are being conducted now. Through population screening there could be a great reduction in the incidence of CF, with carrier couples knowing of their risk before undertaking a pregnancy and in time to opt for termination of an affected fetus. Once the majority of the abnormalities in the CF gene have been discovered, negative screening test results will further reduce the risk of being a carrier to much less than the 1/73, using the single commonest abnormality test that exists now. In some countries with a high frequency of the commonest abnormality in the CF gene, a negative test indicates a risk lower than 1 in 73.

The discovery of the functions of the CF gene may, in time, allow effective treatment to be developed. By then, prenatal testing or detection of those at risk may become less important. Until then, a reduction in the incidence of the disease is the best that the discovery of the CF gene can confer.

FUTURE PROSPECTS

The most important question now that the CF gene has been isolated is how soon it will be before this fundamental advance can be translated into more efficient treatment of CF. Of course, this is an impossible question to answer! However, scientists now have the tools to start designing experiments that will increase our knowledge of how the CF gene works. With increasing understanding of basic mechanisms of CF, direct applications to treatment will undoubtedly be generated. Even though medical science is now reasonably effective at treating most symptoms of CF at least for a certain time period, these treatments are indirect. In other words antibiotics treat bacterial infections to prevent or reduce lung damage, and digestive enzyme supplements partially obviate the need for a functional pancreas. However, these treatments are not directly correcting the CF gene defect itself at the level of the specialized ductal epithelia (see p. 78). Future improvements in treatment will be aimed at achieving this directly.

Two major thrusts in this direction are likely to occur simultaneously. The first will be attempting to use classical pharmacological approaches to correct the CF gene defect. The successful conclusion of this type of approach would be the production of a drug that could directly abolish, or at least substantially alleviate, the damaging effects of having CF. The second approach to correcting the CF gene defect will undoubtedly involve attempts at gene therapy. This rather futuristic term should not generate fear in the reader but merely arouse interest. In this context, the term gene therapy merely describes an attempt to correct the CF gene defect at a genetic (DNA) level. This might either be by replacing the cells in the body that are expressing the basic defect (for example, replacing CF lung epithelium with non-CF lung epithelial cells), or more probably by replacing the CF gene with a non-CF normal counterpart gene in the same cell. Now that the CF gene has been isolated it is possible to start designing laboratory experiments aimed at finding out whether such gene replacement is possible for the CF gene. However, the probability of such an approach being clinically useful is definitely a concept of the future. Even for genetic diseases for which the gene was isolated more than ten years ago, this type of approach to treatment has yet to be achieved successfully. It seems likely that the classical pharmacological pathway may well win the race for effective life-long treatment for CF.

7

Organizations concerned with cystic fibrosis

(A1) THE CYSTIC FIBROSIS RESEARCH TRUST

The Cystic Fibrosis (CF) Research Trust was founded in 1964 by the late John Panchaud, an international businessman whose daughter had CF. Together with Dr Archie Norman (Consultant Physician to John Panchaud's daughter) and Consultant Paediatrician Dr David Lawson, John Panchaud set up the CF Trust in part of his own offices in the City of London.

The objectives of the Trust today are the same as they were when it was founded:

1. To finance research in order to find a complete cure for cystic fibrosis, and in the meantime, to improve current methods of treatment.

2. To form regions, branches, and groups throughout the United Kingdom, for the purpose of helping and advising parents about the everyday problems of caring for CF children.

3. To educate the public about the disease and, through wider knowledge, to help promote earlier diagnosis.

The Trust raises funds continuously for CF research, through national events such as the annual 'CF week' and by the local activities of its regional groups and branches. In fact, since its foundation, the Trust has provided over eleven million pounds towards its objectives. A Research and Medical Advisory Committee, consisting of members of the medical and scientific community, advise on how the Trust can best spend its resources.

The CF Trust's association with local groups is strong. It depends on regional branches and groups for the majority of its income; at the same time it acts as an information source for branches. The Trust produces a valuable regional and branch group manual. This manual covers topics as wide-ranging as how to form and run the branch or group; the officers needed and how meetings should be organized; efficiency in fund-raising activities; publicity for the Trust through local newspapers, radio, and television; and government grants available to CF patients and their families.

(A2) THE NORTH AMERICAN CYSTIC FIBROSIS FOUNDATION [CFF]

The CFF was founded in 1955 to fund research into treatment and cure for CF and to improve the quality of life of individuals with the disease. It currently funds 11 multidisciplinary research centres at universities and medical schools across North America. In addition to supporting basic research and clinical studies, the organization finances more than 120 CFF care centres which provide comprehensive care for those with CF.

The CFF produces brochures and fact sheets on many CF-related topics: for example, health insurance and financial assistance programmes. It also acts as a lobbying body to increase basic science funding and represent the interests of those with CF. The research, medical care, public policy, and education programmes of the CFF are financed by the fund-raising efforts of volunteers at 70 CFF branches and field offices across the USA.

The Canadian Cystic Fibrosis Foundation (CCFF) fulfils a similar role in Canada.

(B) ASSOCIATION OF CYSTIC FIBROSIS ADULTS (UNITED KINGDOM)

The aims and objectives of this association are:

1. To help the CF adult to lead as full and independent a life as possible.
2. To promote the exchange of information.
3. To act as a forum for improving the management of problems encountered by CF adults, both medical and otherwise.
4. To provide encouragement for all those with CF and CF families.
5. To assist wherever possible the efforts of the CF Research Trust.

There is now an active International Association of CF Adults (IACFA).

(C) THE INTERNATIONAL CYSTIC FIBROSIS (MUCOVISCIDOSIS) ASSOCIATION

The International Cystic Fibrosis (Mucoviscidosis) Association (ICF(M)A) was also founded in 1964, on the initiative of the American and Canadian CF Foundations. This organization is an international body, with one national association representing each country. In countries where there is not yet a national CF association, individuals are elected as associate members of the ICF(M)A to represent their countries until a national association has been formed and recognized by the ICF(M)A.

A Scientific and Medical Advisory Council (SMAC), composed of one medical or scientific member from each national association, meets once every four years. This meeting coincides with the major international CF conferences held under the auspices of the ICF(M)A, which bring together the majority of CF research scientists and physicians, a large number of CF allied professionals and lay people. In the intervals between CF congresses, a thirteen-member executive carries out the functions of the SMAC. This executive meets annually in parallel with the European Working Group for Cystic Fibrosis, which provides continuity in Europe between international meetings. In America the annual North American Cystic Fibrosis conference performs a similar function.

Together the ICF(M)A meetings have provided an international forum for the discussion of the personal, organizational, social, and technical problems of CF. Through this organization, the well-established associations have been able to provide help and guidance to new national associations in the process of setting up. This advice has always tried to take into account the different cultural environments operative in different countries. Key factors here are, for example, the level of involvement of the State in medical and social services and research facilities; variations in national wealth and economic priorities in health care; and attitudes to charities, their organizations, and fund-raising activities both within government and in the community at large.

Within these constraints the purposes of the ICF(M)A, in common with those of its affiliated national associations are as follows:

1. The furtherance of the interests of children and adults who have cystic fibrosis. The improvement of medical care available to these people

and of the psychological and social care available to them and their families.

2. The stimulation, support, and advancement of research into the nature, cause, prevention, treatment, alleviation, and cure of cystic fibrosis.

3. The co-ordination of information services and the interchange of information on all phases of cystic fibrosis.

4. To assist in the formation of national associations devoted to cystic fibrosis, where they are required but do not yet exist.

5. The holding of meetings of representatives of government agencies, organizations, and individuals interested in the prevention, treatment, and cure of cystic fibrosis.

There are now some thirty-three countries whose national CF organizations are members of ICF(M)A and about nine others with associate membership. The full addresses of all these associations (correct as of October 1990) are given in Appendix 1.

APPENDIX 1

Officers of the International Cystic Fibrosis (Mucoviscidosis) Association

President: Mr Martin Weibel, Fliederweg 45, 3138, Uetendorf, Switzerland.

Immediate Past President: Mrs Inge Saxon-Mills, Olgiata 15, Isola 31/B, 00123 Rome, Italy.

Vice Presidents: Dr Per Espeli, Klippervejen 4, 3770 Krager, Norway. Mr Ian Thompson, McArthur, Thompson and Law, P.O. Box 3598 Halifax South, Halifax, Nova Scotia, B3J 3J2 Canada.

Treasurer: Mr Henk J. van Lier, c/o Amro Bank, P.O. Box 2059, 3500 GB Utrecht, The Netherlands.

Secretary: Lady Johnson, 3 Lecky Street, Elm Place, London SW7 3QP, UK.

World Health Organization Liaison Officer: Liliane Heidet, 124 Chemin de la Montagne, CH-1224 Chene-Bougeries, Switzerland.

MEMBERS OF THE ICF(M)A, 1990

Argentina

Associacion Argentina de Lucha Contra La Enfermedad Fibroquistica del Pancreas
Mansilla 2814-30'14', 1425 Buenos Aires, Argentina.

Australia

Australian CF Association
P.O. Box 52, Beverley Hills, 2209 NSW, Australia.

Austria

Oesterreichische Gesellschaft zur Bekämpfung der Cystic Fibrose
Obere Augartenstrasse 26–28, 1020, Wien, Austria.

Belgium

Association Belge de Lutte Contre la Mucoviscidose
Place Georges Brugmann 29, 1060 Brussels, Belgium.

Brazil

Assoc. Brazileira de Mucoviscidose
Rua Alvaro Chaves, No. 28, Ap 108, Laranjeiras (CEP 22.231), Rio de
Janeiro, Brazil.

Canada

Canadian Cystic Fibrosis Foundation
2221 Yonge Street, Suite 601, Toronto, Ontario M4S 2B4, Canada.

Chile

Corporation Para La Fibrosis Quistica del Pancreas
La Canada 6506 (i), La Reina, Santiago, Chile.

Colombia

Dr Jorge Palacios
Calle 20 Norte No. 4-45, 20 Piso, Cali, Colombia.

Costa Rica

Asociacion Costarricense de Fibrosis Quistica
APDO, 337, Zona 9 Pavas, San Jose, Costa Rica.

Cuba

Prof. Luis Heredero
Director, Centro Nacional de Genetica Medica, La Habana, Cuba.

Czechoslovakia

Czechoslovakian Cystic Fibrosis Association
Bitouska 1226/7, Praha 4 140 00, Czechoslovakia.

Denmark

Landsforeningen Til Bekaempelse af Cystisk Fibrose
Hyrdebakken 246, DK-8 800 Viborg, Denmark.

Eire

Cystic Fibrosis Association of Ireland
24 Lower Rathmines Road, Rathmines, Dublin 6, Eire.

France

Association Francaise de Lutte Contre la Mucoviscidose
82 Boulevard Massena, Tour Ancone, 75013 Paris, France.

Germany

Deutsche Gesellschaft Bekämpfung der Mucoviscidose E.V.
Adenaueralle II, 5300 Bonn 1, Germany.
  Klinik für Kinderheil-Kunde der Wilhelm-Pieck-Universitat Rostock,
Rembrandtstrasse 16/17 Rostock, 2500 Germany.

Greece

Hellenic Cystic Fibrosis Association
Angelou Sikelianou 8, N. Psychico 15452, Athens, Greece.

Hungary

NWG for Cystic Fibrosis
Department of Pediatrics, Albert Szent-Gyorgyi Medial University,
H-6701, Szeged, P.O.B. 471A-Hungary.

Israel

Cystic Fibrosis Foundation of Israel
Benjaminstr 5, Tel-Aviv 67-4591, Israel.

Italy

Lega Italiana Delle Assoc. per la Lutta Contro la Fibrosi Cistica
Via Seminario n. 10, 30026 Portogruaro, Venezia, Italy.

Mexico

Asociacion Mexicana de Fibrosis Quistica
Altavista Num 21, Col San Angel, Mexico 01000, D.F.

The Netherlands

Nederlandse Cystic Fibrosis Stichting
Lt. Gen. van Heutszlaan 6, 3743 JN Baarn, The Netherlands.

New Zealand

Cystic Fibrosis Association of New Zealand
P. O. Box 18–773, Christchurch 9, New Zealand.

Norway

Norwegian Association for Cystic Fibrosis
P.O. Box 5826, Hegdehaugen 0308, Oslo 3, Norway.

Poland

Polish Society Against Cystic Fibrosis
os. Tysiaclecia 62/64, Krakow, Poland

Portugal

Associacão Portuguesa de Fibrose Quistica
Hospital de Santa Maria, Av. Egas Moniz, 1900 Lisboa, Portugal.

South Africa

National Cystic Fibrosis Association
25 Hope Road, Orange Grove 2192, South Africa.

Spain

Asociacion Espanola Contra la Fibrosis Quistica
Julio Palacios 4, 28929 Madrid, Spain.

Sweden

Swedish Association of Cystic Fibrosis
Box 1827, S-751 48 Uppsala, Sweden.

Switzerland

Schweizerische Gesellschaft fur Cystische Fibrose
Bellevuestr. 166, CH-3028 Spiegel, Bern, Switzerland.

UK

Cystic Fibrosis Research Trust
Alexandra House, 5 Blyth Road, Bromley, Kent BR1 3RS, UK.
Association of CF Adults (UK)
Alexandra House, 5 Blyth Road, Bromley, Kent BR1 3RS, UK.

Uruguay

Asociacion de Fibrosis Quistica del Uruguay
Francisco Rodrigo 2975, Apt 4, Montevideo 11600, Uruguay.

USA

Cystic Fibrosis Foundation
6931 Arlington Road, Bethesda, Maryland 20814, USA.

ASSOCIATE MEMBERS OF THE ICF(M)A

Bulgaria

Dr A. Kufardjieva
Medical Academy, 1st Pediatric Clinic
Georgi Sofiisky Str. 1, 1431 Sofia, Bulgaria.

Finland

Keuhkovammaliitto RRY/CF-Toimikunta, Pohjoinen Hesperiankatu 15 A, 00260 Helsinki, Finland.

Iceland

Icelandic CF Association
Barnadeild Landspitalana, v/Baronsstig, Reykjavik, Iceland.

Japan

Dr Y. Yamashiro
Dept. Pediatrics, Juntendo University School of Medicine,
2-1-1 Hongo, Bunkyo-ku, Tokyo 113, Japan.

Paraguay

Dra L. Garcete de Aguero
Clinica Fleming, Eligio Ayala 1061, Paraguay.

Romania

Dr Popa Ioan
Str. Iancu Vacarescu nr 24, Et. 11, ap. 8, 1900 Timisoara, Romania.

Saudi Arabia

Dr H. Nazar
Dept. Pediatrics, King Faisal Specialist Hospital and Research Centre
P.O. Box 3354, Riyadh 11211, Kingdom of Saudi Arabia.

Turkey

Professor of Pediatrics
Institute of Child Care
Hacettepe University, Hacettepe, Ankara, Turkey.

USSR

Soviet Association for Cystic Fibrosis
Pogodinskaya 8-2, GSP-3 Moscow, USSR.

IACFA

Chairman IACFA
Deurloostr. 5, 1078 HR Amsterdam, The Netherlands.

APPENDIX 2

Glossary

Acidosis — Condition resulting from accumulation of acid or depletion of the alkaline (bicarbonate) reserves in the blood or body tissues.

Aerosols — Medications given by inhalation, usually involving the wearing of a mask over the nose and mouth. In CF antibiotics, bronchodilators, saline, and occasionally mucolytics are given this way.

Alleles — The two forms of the same gene coexisting in the same cell, one being inherited from each of the parents.

Alveoli — Tiny, air-filled sacs in the lung tissue.

Artificial insemination by donor — Insemination of a female with sperm from an unknown donor in a sperm bank instead of that of her partner.

Autosome — All chromosomes other than the sex chromosomes.

Bacteria — Microorganisms (e.g. *Staphylococcus, Pseudomonas*), some of which may invade healthy tissues, others only damaged tissue, to cause infections. Some bacteria, e.g. the *Bacillus coli* of the large bowel, cause no infection and are in fact necessary for health.

Ball-valve effects — These occur in those segments of the lung that have become overdistended through air getting past an obstruction on breathing in, but less getting past on breathing out.

Base — A substance that reacts with an acid to form a salt and water only.

Bronchiectasis — A state of permanent weakening of the bronchial walls, often because of infections and ball-valve phenomena which result in poor drainage of infected mucus.

Bronchioles — Small bronchi.

Bronchodilator — A substance capable of relieving bronchospasm.

Bronchospasm — A reversible spasm (contraction) of the bronchi.

Bronchus (plural **Bronchi**) — Major branch of the airways.

Carrier — An individual who has inherited a particular defective form of a recessive gene from one of his parents, but a normal form from the other. He thus 'carries' the defective gene, but suffers no ill effects from it.

Cholecystitis — Inflammation of the gall bladder, often associated with gallstones.

Chromosomes — The structures within each cell that contain the genetic material.

Cilia — Minute mobile, hair-like processes projecting from the outer surface of a cell. The airways are lined with ciliated cells.

Cirrhosis — Fibrosis of the liver, interfering with the passage of blood from the intestine through liver cells.

Coeliac disease — An inability to digest wheat proteins.

Consanguinity — Inbreeding between genetically related members of the same family.

Cystic fibrosis transmembrane conductance regulator (CFTR) — The protein made by the CF gene. It is thought to regulate movements of charged molecules across cell membranes.

Delta F508 — The common mutation found in 70 per cent of CF genes in Northern Europe and North America. It is caused by the loss of 3 bases in the DNA resulting in the amino acid phenylalanine at position 508 in the protein being absent.

Diploid — Cells carrying two sets of genetic information.

Diuretic — Substance causing the increased production of urine.

DNA (deoxyribonucleic acid) — The major component of the genetic material. The biological molecule that codes for all the information needed to construct a human being from a single fertilized egg.

DNA amplification — A technique for making many thousands of copies of a specific piece of DNA.

Dominant — An abnormal gene, the effects of which are not masked by the presence of its normal counterpart in the same cell.

Duodenal intubation — A process whereby the end of a soft polythene tube is swallowed and passed via the stomach into the duodenum, allowing the contents to be studied chemically, both as regards enzymes and alkalinity.

Emphysema — Permanent overdistension of the alveoli in the lung.

Endocrine glands — These pass their secretions directly into the bloodstream, e.g. insulin and glucagon from the pancreas.

Enema — Injection of liquid into the rectum.

Erythrocytes — Red blood cells, the cells that are responsible for carrying oxygen in the blood and so round the body.

Exocrine gland — A gland that passes its secretions by ducts, e.g. trypsin and lipase from the pancreas. (The pancreas is both an exocrine and an endocrine gland.)

Fibrosis — The replacement of normal tissue with scar tissue, e.g. in the pancreas. Hence the name *Cystic Fibrosis*: fluid-filled cysts develop in the obstructed parts of the pancreas.

Flatus — Breaking of wind.

Genes — Coding regions of DNA.

Genome — All the genetic information of an individual.

Haematemesis — The vomiting of blood. In CF this would most often be associated with cirrhosis and varices.

Haemoptysis — The coughing of blood, usually indicative of advanced CF.

Haploid — Cells carrying one set of genetic information (i.e. eggs and sperm).

Heart–lung transplants — Replacement of heart and lungs of CF patient with those of an organ donor.

Heterozygote — An individual who has inherited different forms of a particular gene from both parents.

Homozygote — An individual who has inherited identical forms of a particular gene from both parents.

Hormones — Specific substances produced in endocrine glands (see above) that are secreted into the blood and are carried to all parts of the body. Hormones are quick-acting, required in very small amounts, and have a wide range of effects on body biochemistry.

Ileus — Literally, a disorder of motility of the ileum, resulting in the contents not being propelled towards the colon. In meconium ileus, contents are not propelled because of the tenacious meconium.

Ileostomy — The bringing of a loop of ileum to open onto the anterior abdominal wall to allow bowel contents to be passed, when there is an obstruction lower down.

Immunosuppressant drugs — Drugs that suppress the natural immunological response of the body to reject foreign tissues and proteins.

Intussusception — A pathological process in which a section of the small intestine closer to the stomach folds into the adjoining region of downstream bowel, endangering its blood supply.

In vitro fertilization — Fertilization of an egg by a sperm in a test-tube in the laboratory.

Ion — An electrically charged atom or molecule.

Isotonic — Having the same electrolytic composition, as do most body tissues.

Lingula — Part of the upper lobe of the left lung.

Malabsorption — Inability to absorb food normally in intestines due to poor digestion.

MCT oil — Oil containing medium-chain triglycerides. These can be absorbed directly into the bloodstream from the intestine.

Meconium — The first dark-green stools of the newborn.

Meconium ileus — An obstruction of the small intestine at birth.

Meiosis — The cell division process by which haploid cells are made from diploid ones.

Mesentery — The membrane carrying the blood vessels to and from the bowel.

Messenger RNA — Copied from DNA by transcription, this molecule is the blueprint for translation of the genetic information into biologically useful molecules, proteins.

Mucolytic — Substance capable of thinning mucus. It may do this by increasing the water content of the mucus or by breaking chemical bonds between sulphur and hydrogen.

Mutation — The occurrence of a spontaneous abnormality in a gene that is not found in the genes of the parent's cells.

Nasal polyp — A growth resulting from the heaping up of mucous membrane in the nostril. Common in older children with CF.

Organ rejection — Loss of function of donor organs due to the new host's immunological response to them.

Osteomyelitis — Infection of the bone, often caused by *Staphylococcus* bacteria, generally in people free of CF.

Pancreatin — Extract of animal pancreas.

Parenteral — Given by a route other than the alimentary canal (digestive system) - usually by vein.

Pathogenesis — The evolution of the abnormal (pathological) changes of a disease process.

Peritoneum — The membrane lining the walls of the abdomen.

Peritonitis — An acute inflammation of the peritoneum.

Phenylketonuria — A genetic disease that results in inability to break down phenylalanine in the diet.

Pneumothorax — Air trapped between the outside (pleural) surface of the lung and the chest wall. This splints the lung and prevents its normal movement during breathing. In CF it would occur with the rupture of overdistended (emphysematous) alveoli. Removal of the air by a needle attached to an underwater drain may be necessary.

Probe — A segment of DNA that is complementary to part or all of the DNA sequence of interest.

Prolapsed rectum — Found in young infants with CF, usually before diagnosis. Malabsorption of fat, with very frequent stools, results in the inner lining of the rectum protruding through the anus.

Proximal bowel — Section of bowel closer to the mouth. (**Distal bowel** — Bowel section further from mouth, i.e. closer to anus.)

Recessive — An abnormal gene, the effects of which are masked by the presence of its normal counterpart in the same cell.

Recombination — The physical process by which new combinations of genes are made by shuffling of the genetic information prior to cell division.

Sclerosing agents — Drugs that strengthen the blood vessel wall.

Spirometer — An instrument for measuring the air breathed into and out of the lungs.

Sputum — Phlegm coughed up from the airway passages.

Steatorrhoea — Literally, fatty diarrhoea. Recognized by pale, bulky, foul-smelling stools.

Steroids — A group of substances that can be natural or artificial and which have a wide range of effects when given as medicines, including suppression of immunological responses.

Varices — Dilated veins.

X-linked — A gene on the X chromosome.

Index